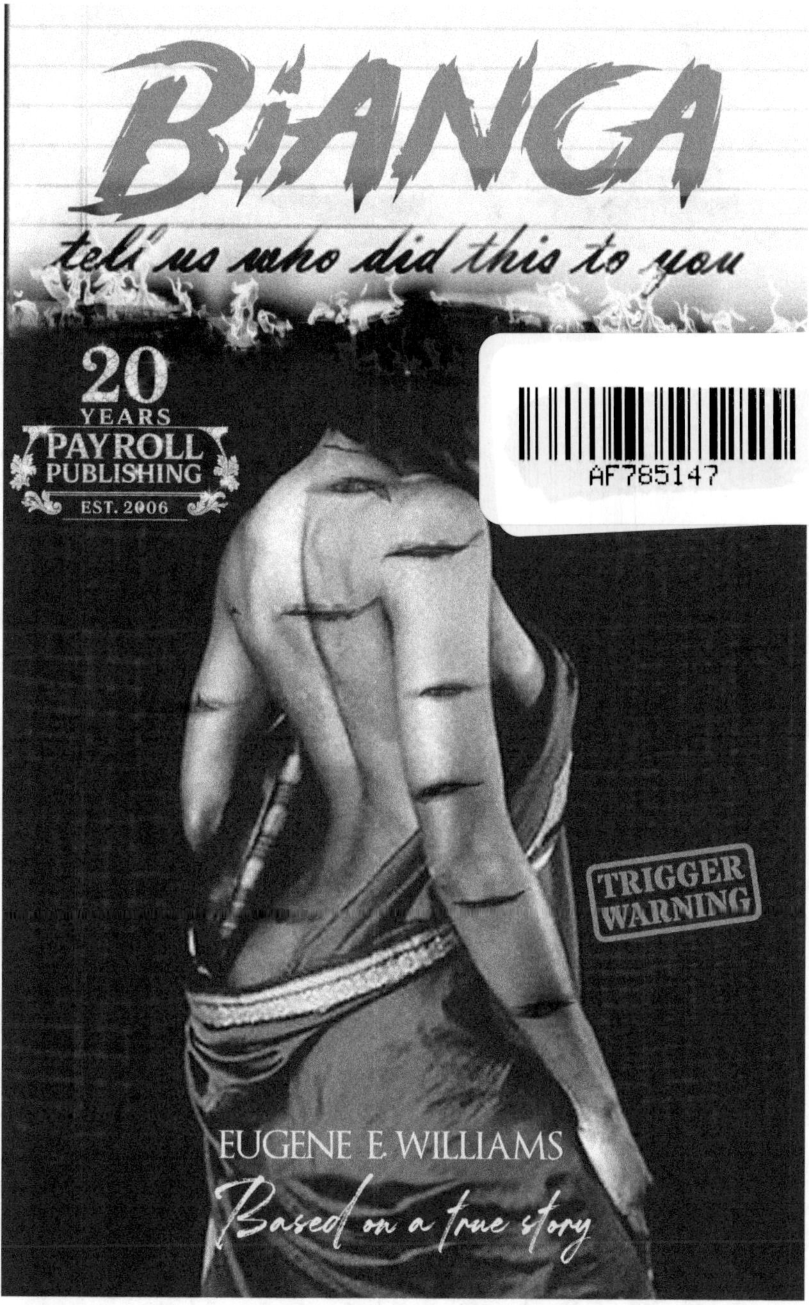
BIANCA
tell us who did this to you
20 YEARS
PAYROLL PUBLISHING
EST. 2006
TRIGGER WARNING
EUGENE E. WILLIAMS
Based on a true story

First Payroll Publishing paperback printing 2006


Published by Payroll Publishing

Library of Congress Control Number: 2007924282



Cover design by M.S. Graphics

For information regarding special discounts for purchases,
please contact,

www.PayrollPublishing.com

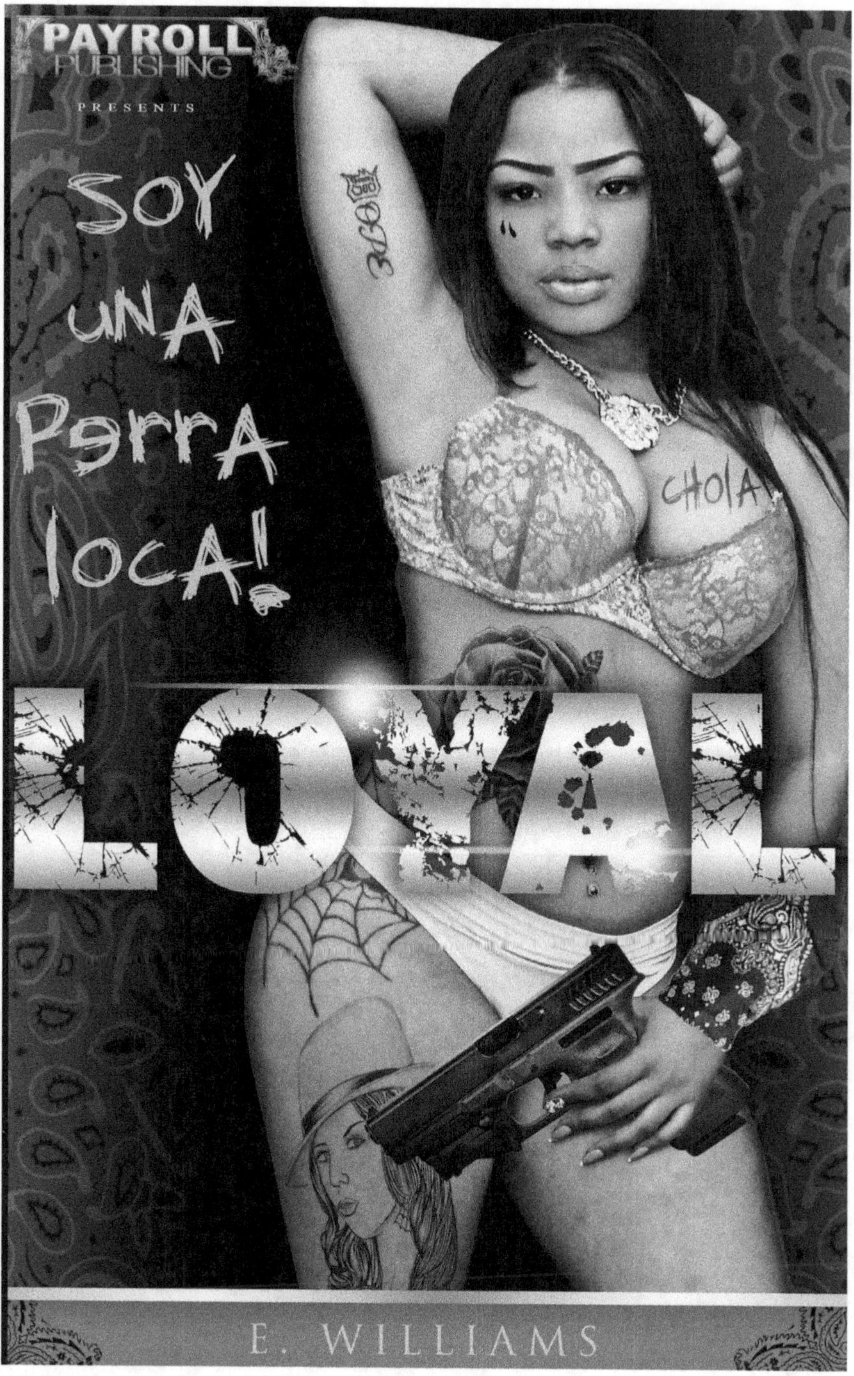
PAYROLL
PUBLISHING
PRESENTS
SOY UNA Perra loca!
CHOLA
LOYAL
E. WILLIAMS

# Table of Content

# BIANCA

*Based on a true story*

**Payroll Publishing**

# TRIGGER WARNING

TRIGGER WARNING: This book contains sensitive material that may be triggering for some readers and survivors of trauma.

The content in this book contains matter that touches on physical and verbal abuse, sexual assault, child abuse, self-injury, suicide, miscarriages, blood, and death.

Practice self-care for mental health wellbeing before, during, and after reading this material.

Reader discretion is advised.

# Chapter 1

# I Remember

At four years old my life seemed normal. But today, I realized my life wasn't normal at all. I'm a twenty-seven year old mother of three. I also have 136 cuts all over my body that happened in one day, and for a long time, I couldn't remember my own childhood. But now I remember everything that happened to me. And it's all because of two terrible situations that happened to my son. One situation happened at church. The other situation, it happened at the church school.

My son Little Keith attended the Pentecostal Church of God Christian Academy. He attended that school because I was raised in that church. The church trained me to raise my children in the way of the Lord, so when they grow old, they won't depart from Him. But one day, I was paid a home visit by a preacher at the church named Evangelist Hart.

And even though I had just talked to Evangelist Hart that past Sunday in service, I didn't expect him to come to my home and pay me an unexpected visit. But strangely enough, there he was.

I answered the door before putting on a sweater to cover the cuts on my body. Normally, I cover up so people won't see any parts of my bare skin. But that time, I was caught off guard. He came in and saw the cuts… but he didn't say anything about it. Instead, he acted as if he didn't notice. But I saw the shock in his face when he looked and tried to play it off. I know he heard all of the bad rumors and gossip floating around the church about me. I figured he thought I was crazy like all the other church members did.

After having a seat, Evangelist Hart told me he was visiting all of the parents who had children in grade K. His reason for the visits were to tell us about how the church believed someone may have been sexually assaulting the kindergarteners at the church school.

"Oh no," I said to myself. I was lost for words. I was mad and my heart was broken at the same time. I felt so hurt knowing somebody may have molested my son at his school. My mind started blaming it on another kid. Or maybe it was a teacher? Either way, how could the school let this happen? At that moment, my suppressed childhood memories came back and hit me dead in the heart, all while he sat there and continued to explain.

He told me how molestation was something big that was happening in our church. He said God wasn't pleased with it and we needed to expose any and all child abusers. Even if they had a title behind their names, like Pastor or Minister. We needed to tell.

"Did something happen to my son at school?" I asked him.

"No, nothing happened to him. But even if somebody has done something to you, then you need to reveal it. You need to tell."

I didn't reveal anything to Evangelist Hart. Instead, I just focused on what he told me. "If it happened to you, then you need to reveal it."

That night, I went to bed and tossed and turned all night long. All I could think about was my son and my own bad childhood. I thought back to when I was four years old and we lived in Jacksonville, Florida. It was on a Sunday, not too long after church service.

I remember myself sitting on a man's lap. The crazy thing about this situation was the fact that, I was in love with this man. But not in love like the way a woman would love a man. I was in love with him because I thought he cared about me the way a father or uncle would. I was raised to care about, love and respect this man because he was the Pastor of our church. But as I sat on his lap, he was rubbing on himself and had my panties pulled down to my thighs. Then, the sick bastard started rubbing himself up and down the upper part of my butt-crack. His name was Elder Roosevelt Thomas.

I used to always go over to his house with him and his wife between church services. They used to call me their "Little girl," their "Baby."

At his house, while I was sitting on his lap, he was rubbing himself in my butt-crack. I turned around and looked to see what he was doing. At the time, I had no idea of what a penis was or even looked like. I was totally innocent and just doing what an older person was telling me to do… an older person who was a Pastor with gray hair. I was taught to be obedient and respect what they said. I had no idea that something was actually wrong.

He gave me a cup and told me to drink my Kool Aid *(it was cherry Kool Aid)*. Then he told me to, "Turn around." When I did, I remember something wet splattering on the upper part of my butt. When it happened, I turned around and looked at him again. He was shaking while holding his penis in his hand. I didn't know what was going on. But now I know. He was masturbating on me.

I was still in the bed when I snapped back to reality. I started wheezing and could barely breathe. I forced myself to get up and get on my nebulizer. I needed some oxygen really badly and I was sweating from the nightmare I'd just had while wide awake.

The next day, I just sat around the house and tried to watch television. But at that point, I was just sitting around remembering. As I sat, I could even remember some things like what I ate before I went to the Pastor's house and what he and his wife gave me for dinner. They gave me macaroni and cheese, collard greens, fried chicken and cherry Kool Aid. The Pastor and his wife had children of their own. But they were all grown up at the time. Therefore, I was the only child there.

As I tried to watch television, I remembered more things, like him having me on his bed while he was trying to penetrate me. It was burning and stinging so bad. He tried to make me count to ten. But I didn't even know how to count all the way to ten. "You just count to ten and it'll be over," he kept telling me while on top of me trying to penetrate. Then he switched up and made me get on top of him.

I remember he had me on top of him and both of us were naked. He was going at it for what seemed to be forever. He was sweating all over me and then all of a sudden, his wife walked in.

I'll never forget the expression on her face when she saw the both of us naked. Her mouth just dropped to the floor as we both looked at her. I was half asleep by that time. My little body was so drained and wore out. But did she help me? No, she just closed the door and left.

But I didn't feel like I needed any help because when she came in, I didn't even reach out to her like, *help me.* I didn't feel like anything was wrong with what was going on. I actually thought it was all normal and okay. Especially with her being his wife and coming in and seeing it. With her being a woman, I really thought everything was fine.

I had to get ready to go back to church. When I was in the bathroom, my vagina was stinging and burning really bad. Now it hurts me to know that I was caring for myself at such a young age. When I look back on it, I'm like, *wow, why wasn't I being protected?* I was thinking I was this big happy girl as I wiped myself with some tissue. I even tried to wet the tissue thinking the water would make it stop burning.

I remember standing on my tippy-toes just to turn the knobs on the sink. That's how short I was. I couldn't even reach the sink. I had to stand on my toes and jump up on the sink to turn on the cold water, not even knowing which one was cold and which one was hot. I turned on the hot water first and got burned when I stuck my hand in it with the tissue. So, I had to throw the first tissue away because it had gotten messed up.

I got some more tissue, ran some cold water on it. When I wiped myself, there was blood on the tissue from him trying to penetrate me. I didn't think anything of it. This was between twelve noon and eight o'clock evening Sunday church services. We went back to church and everything was normal. He even gave me a dollar at the church. Then after church, I went back home with my mother.

My vagina stung as long as I can remember living in Jacksonville. Then the stinging stopped once my mother got married and we moved to Fort Myers, Florida. My mother and everybody who used to babysit me knew they couldn't put any soap, detergent, bubble bath or anything in my bath water because it would irritate me. It would burn so bad. And why was it burning? Now that I'm older, I'm able to put all the broken pieces back together because it's like a puzzle. I understand who I am now and why I was the way I was growing up.

I sat on my lounge chair and remembered all of this and then I started to panic. I paced back and forth around the house for about two hours. My daughters were sleep and my son was at school. I felt like I was going to have a nervous breakdown thinking, *how could this happen?* Even though it happened, I had never faced it in my adult life.

As church people, we believe everything that goes on in church is right. And especially as a child. We were made to walk in a straight line when dealing with or talking about a Pastor, Elder, or Bishop. We were raised to respect church people, and most importantly, the church leaders. *What he's doing is right.*

"Don't tell nobody," he used to tell me. "We have to keep this between us. This is our little secret." He even teased me by asking, "Oh, you gonna tell?"

"No I'm not, I promise," I answered him smiling and laughing, not even realizing that I was being scarred for life.

I'm scarred for life and I don't think the scar can ever be healed. Not through counseling, therapy, or even through church. I think God would have to come down himself and give me a new heart for me to be healed. I do think there is a healing process. But will I ever be healed? I don't think so. A lot of times I'm uncomfortable with being sexual because it makes me remember the things he did to me.

Another memory of mine is being at his house when I was five years old. I have no idea why I was there. But I do know I was actually a little scared this time. Fear had crept in, and I was more aware that something could be wrong.

He drove me to his house one night after church. When he took me in his house, I heard someone yelling and screaming. Another man named Vic McKeever (a member of the Pentecostal Church of God in Jacksonville, Florida) was walking out of the bedroom, and there was a little boy on the bed. I think what made me so scared was, there were two more people there. It was the little boy on the bed who looked like he was around five or six years old, and Vic. What scared me the most was when the little boy started crying. I looked him dead in his face, and still to this day, I don't know who he was. At age 27, it haunts me to wonder, *who was that little boy?*

"Hey Bianca," Vic told me.

"Hey," I answered while scared to death because of the little boy crying in the bedroom. And he wasn't crying a regular cry. It was a painful cry like he was being hurt. Then, Elder Thomas took me over to the couch while talking to me.

"The stuff I do with you, I want you to let Vic do it to you," he explained. "Are you my little girl?" he asked me.

"Yes, I'm your little girl," I answered. What's crazy is, once he started talking to me, I started to feel safe. From his touch, I felt a lot more comfortable. And that's crazy because he was the one who was scarring me for life. And now he's telling me he was going to give me to someone else to let him do to me what he does.

After he gave me to Vic, he told him, "Man she's good too. She's good." Then they both busted out laughing. Vic took me on the screened in porch. There was just enough light coming in to where nobody could see us. Then he pulled out his penis. I instantly noticed that Vic's penis was much bigger than Elder Thomas' and it scared me. But Vic didn't care. He just shoved it in my mouth and made me choke.

I was gagging and choking because it was way too much to be shoving in my little mouth. So, I pulled back. And when I did, he grabbed a wire hanger and told me if I didn't do it, he was going to beat me. He untwisted the hanger, then stretched it out the long way. And every time I stopped sucking, he hit me across my back with the hanger. Therefore, I had to keep sucking. I sucked until he finished.

Then, I started spitting on the floor so much till it was like I was vomiting. I had on a yellow shirt and the semen was all over my shirt. Then he told me to go in the bathroom and clean myself up. When I came back from cleaning myself up, Elder Thomas and Vic made me and the little boy have sex with each other… or at least try to have sex with each other. After that, Elder Thomas and Vic held me down while Elder Thomas stuck a Coca Cola bottle inside me. Then they bent me over and stuck it in my behind.

One Sunday, I was at church and was going to the restroom. The men's and ladies' room both sat side by side. Elder Thomas was coming out of the men's room and saw me. He told me to "Come here." Elder Thomas made me go into the men's room with him. That's where he straight up stood me on the toilet and made me bend over so he could put his penis in my rectum.

It was hurting too bad. So, he put his hand over my mouth and told me, "Shut up! Somebody's going to hear you and you're going to get in trouble for being in the boy's bathroom." I knew my grandmother and mother were going to get me for being in the boy's bathroom. Therefore, I tried my best to keep quiet. But I started crying and couldn't stop. So, he stopped. Then, he made me suck it.

Elder Thomas quickly cleaned himself off and made me wash my hands and face off in the men's room. This situation didn't take long because he was rushing and acting really nervous (probably because of someone coming in). Normally when he molested me, we were at his house where he wasn't nervous at all.

When I walked out of the men's room, an usher was walking out of the church kitchen. Elder Thomas turned around from standing at the sink and started to walk out when the usher saw him.

"I caught her in the men's bathroom. I'm 'bout to tell her mama on her," he told the usher.

"You know better than that!" the usher yelled at me. "Girl I'm about to tell your mama on you! You know you ain't got no business in the boy's bathroom!"

So, they told my mother and grandmother and I had to sit in a corner of the kitchen by myself. Then when I got home, I got a beating for being in the men's room that he pulled me into.

I remember when I was just a little bit older. Elder Thomas dragged me by my right ankle down to the foot of his bed, then put his mouth on my vagina. That was the first time that had happened. It was a really strange feeling to me. His mustache and beard felt like a Brillo pad on my bare skin. He started moving his head from side to side like he was really getting into it. He became so aggressive with it that for the first time, I truly felt the hurt in my heart and I knew what was being done to me was most definitely wrong. At that moment, the room became black to me and it was like I had left my body. After that day, everything went blank and I don't remember any more molesting. That was the day when I suppressed everything.

Right around that time, my mother was telling me, "Don't let nobody touch your private parts." I guess my mother figured *okay, she's six years old, so I guess I can start telling her not to let nobody touch her private parts.* When I was three and four, she must have thought I was too young to be introduced to that. But when she started telling me, I started feeling the hurt. I was feeling like, *oh my God! My Mama is telling me not to let nobody touch my private parts and I'm letting it happen! But I can't make it stop! He's too big! He's too strong! I can't make him leave me alone!*

Not long after that, my mother and I were standing outside of the church one night after an evening service. She was standing next to Elder and Sister Thomas' car while talking to them. She and Sister Thomas were really cool with each other. I was holding my mother's hand real tight and hiding behind her. I wasn't old enough to know how serious child molestation was, but now I was old enough to know what he was doing wasn't supposed to be happening.

"Let me get out of here, I don't know what's wrong with this girl," my mother told Sister Thomas. "She's acting like she saw a ghost or something."

Sister Thomas was trying to talk to me, while at the same time Elder Thomas was telling me to come on his side of the car. While he was talking to me, I was putting my face in the side of my mother's hip.

"You want to go home with me?" he asked. "Come on and go home with me." I knew what was going to happen if I went home with them and I was scared to death. "Do you want to come over? I thought you said you were my little girl?" He was trying to make me feel guilty. But as a child, I was already feeling guilty simply because I didn't want to go.

"Girl what's wrong with you? She's squeezing me so tight," my mother told Sister Thomas. And thankfully, I didn't go with them.

For a long time after that, I thought every man I saw wearing a white wife beater T-shirt was going to get ready to do something sexual to me. That's because those were the T-shirts he wore under his church suits. That was the way he normally presented himself to me, in a wife beater T-shirt.

# Chapter 2

# I Was Better Off

When I was seven my mother married a man from the Pentecostal Church of God named Minister Fred Cooley. He was from our church, but he attended a branch in Fort Myers. So, we moved to Fort Myers, Florida and we lived with him. When they got married, that's when the molestation ended. Even the stinging I kept feeling had stopped. But at that time in my life, I really wasn't thinking about, *hey, I've been molested.* I had suppressed it. But I used to always wonder, *why now all of a sudden, I can put bubbles in my bathwater?*

Thinking back, all of the molestation had taken place between the ages of three and six. And I think if I would've stayed in that city, I would've stayed a victim because the molesters went to our church. The church would have these big meetings and conventions for all of the members in different cities to attend. And even after we had moved, every time Elder Thomas would look at me in those church conventions, I would always be scared of him. I mean really scared of him. And I never gave it any thought as to why I was scared because I had totally blocked it out of my mind.

Even in my teenage years *(around sixteen or seventeen)* I would shake when he would "Praise the Lord" with me.

I would shake and tremble when I would see him in the back area of the Convention Center where the restrooms were. When I spotted him, I would try to wait for him to leave. Or, I would go get one of my cousins to walk in there with me. And at every church convention, he said something to me… every single service. I believe the reason he was doing that was because he was trying to see if I remembered. Or, to make sure we were cool and I wouldn't tell.

Years later when I was eighteen, we were at a church convention and Elder Thomas walked up to me while we were in the kitchen. His wife was a few steps away from us. She was buying something from the scholarship foundation table. That's when he walked up to me and shook my hand.

"Praise the Lord. Girl I ain't seen you in a long time. Hey, why don't you come back to Jacksonville with me to have sex because I haven't had sex in a long time?"

I was eighteen years old at the time and that scared me. I hadn't even thought anything about the fact that he had molested me. I just wondered why would he say something like that to me? Why would he just come at me like that? He's the Pastor and an Elder. He has a position, but that didn't stop him. And when he shook my hand and praised the Lord with me, I tried to pull away. But then he squeezed my hand so tight that he left a bruise on it and his hand print was on my hand.

I was dating a guy named Garry Tucker. When I got in Garry's car, I told him all about it. I also told my mother and she told my aunt who also told Sister Ross (the Bishop's wife). After telling, I had to go have a meeting with Sister Ross. When I told her what happened, she said she was going to make sure Bishop Ross knew about it. But nothing was ever done about it. The situation was treated like, *what the fuck ever*.

A bunch of young men my age from the Jacksonville, Florida church *(about ten of them)* all grew up struggling with their sexuality. Then, after they grew to become young adults, they all turned out to be gay. One day I was talking to a friend of mine named Roy McDougal. Roy's brother is one of the gay guys. We all were on a group call when I broke down crying to them about everything. I had never talked to Roy on that level. But when I told him my story, he was like, "Man! Ain't that a bitch! And you wonder why all these guys turned out to be gay!" Then believe it or not, Elder Thomas' name came up.

When Roy's brother started to tell us why these guys were gay, it went like this:

"Well, who molested him?"

"That person did it to him." It was another young guy who molested him.

"When we were little, this person did it to me first."

"Well, who did it to him?"

"That person did it to him."

"Who did it to that person?"

"Elder Thomas did it to him."

"And that's the person who started everything."

Elder Roosevelt Thomas was the root of it all. And it's crazy and sickening because that motherfucker is still there! Over twenty years later, he is still there! At the same church!

Now that I'm older, I know from experience that I was having orgasms when Elder Thomas was molesting me. Can you imagine what that's like to experience an orgasm at three, four and five years old? Some people say, "No, that doesn't exist." But that's bullshit. I was having orgasms when I was being molested and I always knew that feeling that felt so good to me.

As a little girl, sometimes I would sit on the toilet and try to get that feeling back. I know it's really sickening, but you have to understand, I had been fondled with. I used to think once I got married and started having sex with my husband, the feeling would change to something greater. Then after we had sex, I was like, *wow, there's nothing new.*

*It's that same old feeling.* There was nothing surprising about it because I had been having that same feeling ever since I was a little kid.

Later in my life, there was a time I was performing oral sex on my husband and I just broke out crying. It was like the molestation was happening to me all over again. That's why I say molestation will scar you for life. You think there's a healing point. You even believe there's a healing point. But when you're just about almost healed, there's always something that brings it back up again: especially when you go to the same church where the molester is. Every time someone mentions the Pentecostal Church of God, all I think about is him.

Even when I don't go to church, my family members will come home from church and talk about him. There's a lot of things I don't get because I told my mother this happened to me and she's still cool with him and his wife right now to this day. There's no way one of my kids can tell me they were molested and I'll still be cool with their molester. My mother is in some photos with them at the Bishop's Appreciation and she still talks to them on the phone! I almost hated my mother for that shit. But she can't help it. She's fucked up in the head her damn self and I don't think nobody knows this except for me and God.

Sometimes I think I would've been better off left in Jacksonville with the molester. That's because my life only got harder when my mother got married. I was always in a domestic violent and child abusive situation in my home and my own mother wasn't doing nothing about it. So, I started thinking there was nothing to be done about it. I went from being molested, to being abused… me and my little brother.

Just before my mother got married, there was another man in the picture named Bonnie Barker from Winter Haven, Florida. To me, her marriage didn't seem to be too sacred or serious because my mother allowed me to make the choice of which man she was to marry.

"Which one should I marry, Bonnie or Minister Cooley?" she asked me. I chose Minister Cooley because I didn't want to live in Winter Haven. It was a place nobody wanted to be. We hated Winter Haven growing up as kids. We stayed at the church motel during church conventions and the motel was some real bullshit.

I remember the first time Minister Cooley beat me. I was only eight years old. It was as if he already had it out for me anyway. I sensed that he wanted to beat me for a long time. Have you ever felt like somebody just wanted to do something to you, like you know this person wanted to fight you? That's how big of a grudge he had against me.

We were in a church convention called the Bishop's Council. During that convention we were staying at the Holiday Inn. My mother left me and a few of my cousins in the room so Minister Cooley could watch us. He was telling us to stop making noise, and to stop playing, and for me to pick up something from under the table. We were doing what he said and while doing it we were still laughing but not as loud. Then he got a belt that he worked in which had cement and plaster matted on it, and without a warning, he started beating me.

After the beating, I had bruises all over my entire body. I thought he was way out of line for beating me the way that he did while my mother wasn't there. Plus, he wasn't my real father. He was only my step-father. That was my first beating. And as time went on, me, my little brother and my mother all got beatings.

My little brother was only four years old and he wasn't Minister Cooley's son either. But one day we were at the laundromat and Minister Cooley and my mother got into a fight. He picked her up and tried to put her in the car. She busted her ear because he tried to throw her in while she was struggling. When he got her in, he walked to the driver's side of the car, then she got out of the car and started walking. He started driving all wild and crazy to catch up with her. Then, she broke out running. Minister Cooley pulled alongside of her and hit her with the car. All of this was traumatizing to us two young kids in the back seat.

My little brother Deon had his hands on his ears screaming with his face in my lap. I was rubbing his back and telling him everything was going to be okay. From that day on, it was like I became his protector from everybody in the family because they were just so weak. They were so weak till it fucked them up really bad.

Not long after that, my mother and Minister Cooley were in their bedroom arguing and fighting. I came out of my room and saw a bloody knife on the table. And from all of the loud arguing, I became scared. But even as a child, I had to think, and think quickly.

I went into my room to plan out something to do. Because I saw the bloody knife on the table, I wondered, *what can I do to make this stop*? So, I started screaming really loud until the both of them ran into my room.

"What's wrong?" they asked.

"Grandma! Its Grandma!" I screamed.

"What?"

"Grandma, I think she's dead!"

"What are you talking about?"

"I just had a dream and Grandma is dead!"

I was making it up just to get the two of them to stop fighting. And it worked. They called my grandmother for me. Then they went back into the room like two civilized people. Minister Cooley grabbed the knife off the table and took it into the kitchen on the sly like I didn't see it. But I had already seen it.

As I was growing up, me and Minister Cooley didn't get along at all. How could I get along with a man who had the title of a Minister and I constantly saw him fighting and beating on my mother?

There was another situation where he was beating her so bad that it sounded just like it does when a person gets punched on TV. I was hearing the punches come out of their bedroom. Their bedroom door had a square hole in the center with a curtain on it. I pulled the curtain back and he had my mother by her hair punching the shit out of her. And as he was punching her, blood was flying out of her mouth.

I was scared to death when I saw what was going on. So, I ran out the front door then started running down the street. As I was running, Minister Cooley ran out the house yelling, "Bianca! Where are you going?" but I kept running and didn't look back.

I ran to some church people's house that was not too far from our house and told them, "If they come looking for me, tell them I'm not here!" Then I hid in their closet and stayed there. Eventually my parents came over and I had to leave. As they drove me back home, they told me they were sorry. Even when we arrived home, we sat on the couch and he said he was sorry and it wouldn't happen again. I just sat there and cried because I had just seen my mother get her faced bashed in. He told me it wouldn't happen again, but that was some bullshit because it continued to happen, over and over again. Then, we'll go to church and he'll preach about the Lord this and Lord that.

How can he get up and talk about the Lord when he can't even control his own self? He was the most violent person that I had ever seen at that point. And I'm not talking about the little violence they show on TV with these women getting slapped and pushed around. That's not domestic violence to me. What I'm talking about is a man knocking my mother's teeth out with his fist to the point where she had to get dentures at a young age.

I'll never forget one day I walked into the bathroom and my mother was standing at the sink crying while holding her lip up. When I looked at her, it scared the hell out of me because her face was all black and blue. Her teeth were gone and blood was all over the sink and floor.

"Mom, are you okay?" I asked when I walked in.

"GET OUT!" she yelled then slammed my finger in the door. "Get out of here! Get out! Don't come back in here no more, get out!"

I was only trying to help her. But situations like that have me traumatized still to this day. Every time I think about it, it's like, *what the hell? There's not that much forgiveness in the world! But for some reason she's still with him.* I know the truth about everything that has happened. She knows the truth, and he knows the truth. Maybe that's the reason why Minister Cooley can't look me in my face still to this day.

Deon was seeing all of this traumatizing shit as well and he would wet his bed because of it. Every time he would wet the bed, Minister Cooley would tell him he was going to wake him up with a belt and beat him.

Minister Cooley got up for work at five a.m. Then, he would go into my little brother's room to check on him. Naturally, my brother wet the bed because he would go to sleep in fear because they were arguing, fighting, throwing stuff, busting glass and outside breaking windshields. And all while he's in his room trying to go to sleep by himself. So as early as five in the morning, Minister Cooley just started beating him. He didn't even wake him up first. My little brother got woken up with the belt, and then he had to take a bath and go back to bed.

When Minister Cooley would go to work, I would let my little brother come into my room and I'd put peroxide on his cuts. He was being beat so bad to where his skin was ripped open and he was bleeding all over the place. My mother and brother were afraid of Minister Cooley. But at that time, I wasn't and he knew it. Since I wasn't afraid of him, it was like I became his main target.

I felt like I had to protect my little brother because he was so young and helpless, a victim. All throughout middle school and some of high school I would stay awake for as long as I could, playing my keyboard and writing songs until it was time for me to go to school. Sometimes I would stay awake for two and three days because I was trying to protect my little brother. If I did sleep it was only for thirty minutes to an hour. Then, I would get up and put my little brother on the toilet so he wouldn't wet the bed.

I used to tell my cousins and other family members about some of the things that went on in our house. But nobody ever believed me. That's until a couple of my cousins stayed over one weekend and my parents started fighting while we were sitting in the living-room. Minister Cooley was dragging my mother from the kitchen through the dining-room to the living-room, beating her silly.

Even after that, Minister Cooley would complain to my grandmother about me.

"Bianca is just disrespectful," he complained. "She's just rude. She don't wanna listen to me because I'm not her real daddy. She don't have no respect for me."

They would sit right at the dinner table and talk about me in front of the whole family. So after that, I had to hear it from everybody in the family. When we went to church, my uncles looked at me mean. One of my self-righteous uncles pulled me aside and said, "You need to listen to what your step-daddy say! Y'all ain't even his kids! At least you could respect a man in his house!"

They didn't know shit! All of them were on the outside looking in. Let somebody bash their mother's head in and see if they're going to respect that motherfucker. That's why people shouldn't judge other people's situations. If you are not in it, then shut the fuck up!

Eventually, the whole family found out that Minister Cooley was beating my mother. One day my grandmother and my aunt were over when they broke out fighting again. They were in their bedroom where he was beating her and she started screaming out to her mother and sister, "Mama! Mama! Donna! Donna!"

My aunt was getting up to go into the room and help her when my grandmother stopped her.

"You can't help her because she don't want to help herself," my grandmother told my aunt. "She act like she so in love with this man, but she in love with his money."

And that was that. They didn't do anything about it. They felt like she was staying with a man who was dogging her, beating her like crazy, mistreating and beating her kids, and she was with him because he made good money. And maybe they were right.

I should hate my mother for letting us grow up in that bullshit home. It was enough for me to walk away and hate her for the rest of my life. But I don't because she's my mother. So, that's how we lived and it was… some real bull shit.

# Chapter 3

## He's Out To Get Me

There was a time when Sister Green came to Fort Myers, Florida to run a church meeting. Sister Green had a high position in the church. She was the national supervisor of the Women's Department for the Pentecostal Church of God. On the Saturday of the meeting, the women were going to go out and sell Krispy Kream donuts for the scholarship foundation. That morning, Minister Cooley came into my room to wake me up.

I was lying there in a slip and my breast was out. He woke me up by feeling on my breast. Of course, he denied it. But, he did it. I'm a light sleeper and anything wakes me up. Especially, somebody touching me. He reached out and felt on my breast… but I was made out to be a liar by my mother and him. When I opened my eyes and saw him touching my breast, he jumped back and tried to act like he was touching my shoulder. "Bianca, Bianca, wake up," he tried to play it off.

After I got up and dressed myself, I went to the church. Sister Green noticed that I was mad as hell, so I told her what happened. She then told the Pastor, who at the time was a man named Elder Conner. The pastor told Bishop

Ross, who's the Bishop of District #4 *(The Pentecostal Church of God in Florida and California)*. Bishop Ross called me, my mother and Minister Cooley into his office. And this was the day my mother put something between us that can never be moved.

"Is this so, did this happen?" Bishop Ross asked me.

"Yes Sir Bishop Ross," I answered.

At that time, I had so much respect for the "Man of God" that I wasn't about to lie to him. Bishop Ross was a highly respected man. He had grey hair, a long grey beard, and a big stomach like Santa Claus. What he said was law because we thought God spoke to us through him. I was an impressionable teenager back then and everybody was telling me, "You don't lie to Bishop Ross. He knows when you're lying." So, I told him the truth.

"Bianca, I did this to you? Elder Cooley asked me. You're lying! I didn't do anything to you!"

"Okay, but you did it though."

"I don't think she'll keep saying you did if it's not true," Bishop Ross jumped in and commented. "Why would she keep saying you did it?"

I was not about to let it go. I was not about to leave out of there saying he didn't do it because he was trying to overpower me as an adult. An adult trying to out-talk a kid, that's easy. But fuck that, motherfucker you did it! But he was so persistent on saying he didn't do it. And this is what made me have a problem with my mother because she straight up jumped to his defense when we were going back and forth,

"No I didn't!"

"Yes you did!"

"No I didn't!"

"Yes you did! I ain't changing because it's the truth!" The truth is just the truth and you can't change the truth. I didn't want it to be true. But it was true! You think I wanted something like that? Hell naw!

Then after our office meeting, I had to go back home and live with his domestic violent ass! Do you know how scared I was of going home that day?

"I know I'm gonna get a whipping when I get home," I told Bishop Ross.

"For what?" he asked me.

"For telling the truth."

"Don't beat her when you get home, Bishop Ross told him. "Ain't nobody gonna give you a whipping." *That's what you think*, I sat there and thought to myself. "Well Sister Cooley, what do you think about this?"

"I think she's lying!"

When she said that I thought to myself, *motherfucker, this is your chance to tell, not only what he did to me, but what he's done to you!* She was two-faced because she would get in the car with me and tell me about how she was leaving him.

"One day he's gonna come home and we'll be gone!" I was happy because she was finally talking about leaving that abusive motherfucker. "Old black bastard," that was her favorite thing to call him. "You black bastard!"

We were talking about how we were going to get away. Now, you get in the office and switch up on me! If that was today, I would've hit her. God forbid, I would've tried to knock the shit out of my own mama. She chose a man over her daughter. She chose what he had to say over what I was telling her, which was the truth!

"Why do you think she's lying?" Bishop Ross asked my mother.

"Because she can't stand him. She doesn't like him because he's not her real daddy."

Right at that moment, I closed up and wouldn't tell anything else. I went into a shell because I felt betrayed by my own fucking mother. Bishop Ross kept talking to me, but I wouldn't respond.

"Bianca if you don't talk to me, I can't help you."

*Talk to you for what?* I looked at it as if my own mother didn't have my back, then who was going to protect me? If she didn't believe me, then why would he? Who in the fuck was there for me to depend own? Just thinking back on it, I hate my mother for that. She could've saved me from so much other stuff that went on after that.

When we got back home, everything seemed like it was so bad. I was going to school every day straight up not even wanting to live and praying something bad happened to me. I felt worthless, like what's the point of me being here? I had some crazy love for God, but there were times I felt like even he had betrayed me. I felt like he had forsaken me. *How do you allow this Lord? I guess the Lord won't put nothing on me that I can't bear,* I thought to myself.

After that, the verbal and physical abuse towards me became worse. The man had it out for me. Some of the names he called me were a failure and a whore. He'd call me a whore straight up in front of everybody in the house. "She ain't gonna be nothing but a hoe!" But why did I have to be a hoe? I guess because I wouldn't let him touch my breast.

My grandmother once told me, "The only reason he didn't take it no further was because he knew you would tell. It's because of your mouth. You always had a big mouth." If I hadn't opened my big mouth and said something that same morning it happened, only God knows what he would've tried to do to me. If I would've acted scared when I looked into his eyes, he probably would've started raping me. There were many nights when I had to sleep fully dressed in that uncomfortable house.

I used to run away from home to my boyfriend Garry Tucker's house. I would tell him about the things I was going through. But that was unnecessary because he could always see the bruises on my body. One day we were at church and he saw a bruise on my leg and asked, "Did Minister Cooley do that?" I had bruises all over me but he could only see the ones on my leg. I showed him my arm and he said, "Minister Cooley needs his ass kicked!"

Then, people started seeing for themselves how the man hated me. We were at choir rehearsal one day and they claimed I was the best singer in the church. I normally sang soprano. But that day I was asked by the choir director to sing alto. So, I did what I was asked to do. Minister Cooley was in the back of the church with the Brothers watching everything.

"I can't hear y'all!" the choir director shouted. "Sing louder! Sing louder!"

Next thing I knew, Minister Cooley walked up and pushed me in my back, straight up in the church in front of everybody.

"You ain't singing!" he shouted.

"I am singing! She told me to sing alto!" Then he pushed me to the floor so hard that I sprung my arm and busted my fucking mouth. Right in the fucking church, abuse was happening. All those fucking church people were sitting right there and not a damn thing was done about it. That was some real bullshit.

After throwing me to the floor, he took me outside. My nose was bleeding, the top of my lip was busted, my fucking arm was sprung, and I had a knot on my head. He told me he was sorry and a bunch of other bullshit. Then he started talking about the Lord.

"I'm not always right, but the Lord wants to use you. You got a beautiful voice and can sing better than anybody in that church. You can out-sing all those people in there and I know you can sing louder than that. But I didn't hear her tell you to sing alto."

I don't even know how he knew the difference between soprano and alto. He wasn't a singer, but he was acting like he knew. Then, he made me go right back to my same spot and sing in front of everybody, while another motherfucker brought me some ice for my lip.

I was so embarrassed and humiliated. And from that day on, our personal business was just out there. Everybody knew that our house was a dysfunctional home. "Minister Cooley is beating on Sister Cooley," was what the church people said amongst themselves. Then, they started having sympathy for me. But I was still living in a house with a man who hated me.

He was out to get me and he couldn't stand my popularity. He couldn't stand how I was so outgoing. He couldn't stand the fact that every man in the church wanted to fuck me. Every boy wanted to fuck me. Every man we passed in the street wanted me. Man… looking back, I was beautiful! But at the time, my self-esteem was low. I really didn't know what I was yet. I was beautiful and didn't know it.

♫ ♫ ♫ ♫ ♫

My mother and Minister Cooley had two more children while I was a teenager. He never abused his real kids because they were his pride and joy.

I'll never forget the day when he took my baby brother Derrick *(his son)* and held him in front of me and Deon after cussing and fighting with our mother and beating us. "You see this?" he shouted. "This is my son! This is my blood! I'll never love y'all the way I love my own!"

Ain't that some shit to say to some kids? You should never say something like that to some kids. At the time, he had just been promoted to Pastor of the church in Plant City, Florida. He was no longer Minister Cooley. Now he was

Elder Cooley and he called himself a "Man of God" while making a division in his home.

One day I couldn't take it anymore and ran away from home again. I went back to Garry's house. Not long after I got there, my parents came looking for me with the police. Garry's parents (*Deacon and Sister Tucker)* my parents, plus Garry and I were all standing on the porch while the police were talking to me.

"You know what we do to runaways?" the police asked me.

"No Sir, I don't know."

"We take them to a children's home. You'll have to live in a foster home. But this is your choice. You can go home to your beautiful family and your bed… or, get in the car with us then go downtown and get put in a home. We'll book you in and sign you over to the State."

I had a choice to make. Either go back home with Elder Cooley and my mother, or go with the police. Which one do you think I chose? It was scary seeing the police and the red and blue lights flashing from the police car. But I still jumped in the back of the police car.

"Something must be really wrong with this home if this child doesn't want to go back," the officer commented. Even they could see it.

No child is going to jump in the back of the police car instead of jumping in the back of her parent's car! *Fuck that, take me to jail,* was what I was thinking.

"She think she's grown, take her to jail!" my mother yelled. "Scare her up and let her see what it's like! She wanna act like she grown! She wanna jump in the back of the police car and go with y'all, then take her!" My mother and Elder Cooley were telling the officers to rough me up and take me through a bunch of bullshit.

"We're going to make it to where she wants to go home," one officer said. "Let me show you what happens to young people like you."

After that, they drove off with me in the back seat. "What's going on in your home that you don't want to go back?" the officer asked. I didn't even answer the officer's question. And in fact, I should've been scared to death. But I wasn't. I felt good and safe in the back of that police car like a criminal.

At that age, I had a lot of respect for the police and didn't know anything about corrupt cops or police brutality. All I knew was when I saw the police, they were coming out to my school talking about, "Officer friendly. We're there for you when you're in trouble." Well, take me wherever y'all have to take me, but please don't take me back to that house because there's trouble there.

In the back of that police car, I exhaled for the first time in a long time. I was happy and tears of joy were rolling down my face.

The police took me to the so-called rough side of Fort Myers, Florida named Anderson, then later renamed Martin Luther King Boulevard. We went to some abandoned homes where people were smoking crack. As they were walking and talking to me, I was trying my best to only tell the police certain things I wanted them to know. I knew if I told them everything, they were going to take my mother's kids away from her.

"You don't want to end up like this. You don't want this type of life for yourself, do you?" the officers asked.

"Naw, I don't want that," I answered as they pointed out some prostitutes.

"These women get beat up out here. You don't want to experience that."

"Well, I've already experienced getting beat up."

"Who beat you up?"

I messed up and said too much. And at that point, I stopped talking. "We can't help you if you don't talk to us." The officer zipped up my jacket then squatted on his knees. "Honey, we're here to help you. If something's going on in your home… Well, I know it's something going on in your home for you to choose to come with us instead of going with your mother. Was she your real mother?"

"Yes, she's my real mother."

"Is that your real father?"

"No, he's my step-father."

"Tell me, I know something is wrong."

I didn't tell him anything, so they took me to a girl's home. In the girl's home, I was very anti-social and kept my distance from the other girls. There was a piano there, so I sat at the piano and started playing. I loved music and played by ear without ever being taught. Then before I knew it, all eyes were on me.

"Oh, she plays the piano," one of the women who worked there blurted out. "Honey, you have such a big future ahead of yourself. You're going to be successful one day."

Everybody who met me believed I was going to be successful in my music career. "You're so talented. You're so gifted." Playing the piano helped me to open up and be more social to the people there. I told them how I learned to play and what church I went to. And eventually, the woman talked me into going back home.

"I bet your little brother misses you," she told me and "brother" was the key word.

I went back for Deon, and he probably never knew it. When she mentioned him, my heart started beating fast and I thought, *damn I left him!* Then, I started thinking about the horrible things Elder Cooley could've been doing to him. So, I went back feeling like I couldn't be broken.

♫ ♫ ♫ ♫ ♫

By the ninth grade, I was attending the school of the arts and was making good grades. Me and a close friend used to sign people's year books *(even though we were freshmen)* because they just knew we were going to be famous one day.

The seniors told me if I wasn't going to be a singer, then I was going to have my own talk show. They just knew I was going to be something great. But now look at me. I'm a nobody, trying to tell everybody about the bullshit I've been through.

One day after school I was doing my homework and listening to the air-conditioner rattle our old window. All of a sudden, I heard a loud "Boom!" The first thing I thought was my mother's mirror fell off the dresser because it wasn't attached all the way. I didn't hear any yelling or fussing, so that's what I thought. I ran into her bedroom and before I could say 'are you alright,' Elder Cooley had my mother on the floor punching her. Soon as he saw me open the door, he picked up his tennis shoe and threw it in my face as hard as he could. "Get the fuck out!" he screamed at me.

He had told me before if they were ever fighting, I better not ever come in and try to help my mother. I was younger when he told me that. It was right after they had finished fighting and I ran in the room screaming, "Stop! Stop! Leave my mama alone!" We all sat down to talk about what they were acting stupid over when he told me that bullshit right in front of her.

"We're grown and if you ever see us fighting, you just stay out of it."

"Yeah Bianca, you just stay out of it," she co-signed.

Elder Cooley hit me in my face with his shoe so hard that the next morning I went to school with his shoe print on my face. By that time, I'd seriously had enough. When I arrived at school, I wrote my vocal assemble teacher a letter saying how my mom and step-father were fighting all night and I didn't get any sleep. I asked if she could please excuse me because I wanted to lie down and get some rest because I was tired and sleepy.

Before I knew it, I was called down to the office and the Social Service had gotten involved. Social Services called my mother and told her they were coming to check her home to make sure her kids weren't being abused. I was scared as hell and thought I was really going to get in trouble because my mother was going to get her kids taken away.

When I got home, my mother and Elder Cooley were fussing and fighting again because of the letter I gave to my teacher. I stayed in my room that whole day, then went back to school that next morning. That afternoon, while sitting in class, I got an emergency phone call on the classroom phone from my mother.

"Um, hello?" I answered after my teacher gave me the phone.

"Bianca, I hope you're happy!" my mother yelled. "I hope you realize what kind of damage you did! I knew this was what you wanted all along! Thanks to you, these people are coming to take my kids! They taking you, they taking all my kids away from me!"

"But Mama, it did happen."

"It's all because of what you wrote in that letter and what you told them!"

"But Mama, it really happened. It happened."

Throughout my life, my family had me believing and feeling like I was the sick person: like I was the one with the problem, and I was the crazy one: when all along they were the sick individuals. Do you know how crazy that is when you're living with some dysfunctional people and they're trying to make you out to be the one who's crazy?

But my mother was on the phone crying and straight up flipping out.

"I hope you're happy! If I can't have my kids, then it ain't no reason for me to live! I'm just gonna go and kill myself! I'm committing suicide!"

"No Mama!" I screamed, alerting all the other kids in the classroom.

"I want you to know, I'm going to just kill myself! I'm just gonna go and jump off a bridge! I'm going to kill myself! I hope you're happy! You won't have to worry about me, you won't have to worry about him! You'll have a new mama and a new daddy!"

After she told me she was going to kill herself, I ran and grabbed my backpack and told my friend David to drive me home. By that time, the Dean and all of the other school officials were looking for me. They saw me running down the hall and yelled out for me. But I kept running. Then I was cut off by the assistant principal before I ran out of the door.

"Bianca calm down!"

"No, I gotta go home! My Mama finna kill herself! I gotta go home!"

It was the worst feeling in the world, to be sitting in my classroom and get a call from my mother saying she was about to kill herself. I felt like if I didn't get there in enough time, she was going to be dead. All I was thinking was, when I got home, she was going to be dead. But when I made it home, she was okay. Every time I think about that situation, it does something to my insides.

A woman from the church came over to stay with my mother for a while and I ended up going to her house. While I was there, my mother called me and said the only way they weren't going to take her kids was if I go back to school and tell them I lied.

"Well… I know it's true," my mother told me. "You know it's true. But what goes on in this house stays in this house."

That was some bullshit! Some of the things that went on in our house didn't need to stay in our house. Shit needs to be revealed or else you'll have people like me who grow up and be scarred for life.

So, I had to go back to school and say I lied. I had to ruin my reputation with the school officials. We had to sit in a meeting with some social workers and I had to make up a big lie so my mother could keep her kids. I had to sit there and get chewed out by this one social worker.

"Bianca, it's not good for you to make up things like this! You could've had your mother in a whole lot of trouble because the State was ready to come in and take all of you away!"

I was feeling like shit because I thought I was ruining my reputation at the school. The entire staff knew me and they didn't think I was a bad person up until that point. When we walked out of the meeting, the head principal tapped me on my shoulder and said, "Bianca it's going to be okay. I know you weren't lying. If you ever need somewhere to go, here's my number." My teacher just looked at me as if she also believed me. That made me feel so good and tears filled my eyes. "If there's one thing we know you're not, we know you're not a liar."

To live in that domestic violent and abusive home was hell enough. And for my mother to make me out to be a liar when the shit was really happening was even worse. They stood before the church people and the "Man of God" and said it didn't happen. And for somebody to believe me was all I wanted in the first place.

Right after that, my teacher came over to our house and had a talk with me and my mother.

"Bianca is such a good student and such a good girl. We don't have any problems out of her and everybody loves her. Bianca is very popular and so smart. She's so gifted and talented. Do you know how good your daughter can sing? Bianca is going to be famous and we're going to be watching her on TV one day."

There were a bunch of positive things she told my mother and it was like, *so what*. What my teacher said about me didn't mean shit because the house was too dysfunctional for anybody to notice that, *hey, Bianca is talented, or Bianca is gifted. She's going to be a star and be on TV one day.*

♫ ♫ ♫ ♫ ♫

There was another situation that happened when I was between fourteen and fifteen years old. I had gotten pregnant by Garry. When my mother and Elder Cooley found out, I was already three months into the pregnancy. They had Garry come over and we all had a meeting in the living room. They asked us what we were going to do about the situation and was he going to be there for the baby?

"Bianca, what are you going to do?" Elder Cooley asked me.

"I'm going to take care of it."

I didn't know what was wrong with what I said, but what else was I supposed to say? Whatever the case was, Elder Cooley snapped on me.

"You better be glad your ass is pregnant because I would've knocked you out of that chair! With your smart-ass mouth, 'I'm gonna take care of it!'"

But what was I supposed to say? I didn't even say it in a nasty way. And even if I did, the point I'm trying to make is that I couldn't say anything and win. I was living in a house with a man who hated me and he was out to get me.

I had already revealed how he tried to touch my breast. So, any little thing I said or did was bad to him because I was his target.

After our meeting, I went to school every day as normal. At that time, I was being mistreated by a prejudiced teacher. He smoked weed and bought it from the high school students. I got an A in all my other classes. But this one teacher gave me an F on my report card. I told my mother about the guy and she came up to the school to see what was going on. She had already known he was a jerk and she wanted to see if he was really giving me a hard time.

So, one day I walked into the classroom and he just told me to "Get out!" It was for no apparent reason. I wasn't late or anything. So I just looked at him like, *I'm not going nowhere,* then I sat down in my chair.

"I told you once and I'm not going to tell you no more!" Everybody in the class was like, *damn, what did she do?* I hadn't even given the man any problems or anything. I wasn't getting crunk in the class or nothing. I took my math book out like, *this motherfucker don't tell me to get out. This is where I'm supposed to be this class period.*

"Get out!"

"No."

"I'm going to write you up! I don't want you in my classroom!"

I was pissed at that point because he was just picking on me. So I got up and walked over to his desk.

"You know what, I'm going to get out. But before I go, write on my referral that I called you a **BITCH!** because that's what you are, you a motherfucking **BITCH!** You ignorant ass motherfucker! You probably can't even spell the shit!"

I cussed his ass out and was I wrong for doing it. Disrespecting my elders was something I didn't do. But I didn't give a fuck at the time. Then, when he gave me my referral, I ripped it up and threw it. The classroom started hollering, clapping, banging on the desks yelling, "Whooo whooo whooo! Biancaaaa! As I walked out of the class, I heard them say, "I told you she was a church girl! She ain't wit that shit!"

By the time I got home, the school had called and left the whole situation on the voice mail for my mother to hear. Elder Cooley heard it first. And by him hearing it first, God forbid what happened to me next.

"Bianca, did you call your teacher a bitch and tell him to make sure he spell it right?" he asked me soon as I walked through the door.

"Yes Sir," I answered.

"Why?" I started to tell him why, but he cut me off. "You know what? I don't even wanna hear it damn-it! You don't be out to that school talking to those teachers any kind of way! I'm gonna beat your behind before your mama gets here. I know she's not gonna want you to get it because you're pregnant! But as far as I'm concerned, I don't give a damn about you, or that baby! You can fuckin' lose it for all I care! Go get in a slip! Come out your clothes, get naked and get in a slip!"

At that time, I didn't even know he could have gone to jail for beating me while I was pregnant. But when I changed into my slip, he just beat me and beat me, then beat me some more, and I was pregnant… We had sat there and had a meeting with Garry and everything, but he still beat me… He beat me so bad to where I felt a pull in my stomach that hurt so bad it made me fall to the floor. When I hit the floor, blood started running down my legs.

While I was on the floor, he took the belt that was wrapped around his hand and wrapped it in the opposite direction exposing the buckle. At that point, he couldn't see the blood. He told me to "Get up!" And when I got up, he swung the belt and hit me dead in my eye with the buckle. That was my first black eye ever.

I ended up at the hospital that night. Then I had a miscarriage and lost the baby that same night. Fresh bruises were all over my body because I was severely beaten not too long ago.

"Honey who did this to you?" all the nurses asked. I didn't talk to anybody. Instead, I turned over on my stomach, laid there and cried. I knew if I talked, they were going to come and take my mother's kids away from her. I didn't talk so she could keep her kids.

Every time somebody came into the room, they asked me who did that to me. One nurse would go and get another nurse, "Look at this," they said while showing the bruises on my back, arms, and legs, plus my black eye. One of them even had tears in her eyes, but they didn't roll down.

"Honey, we want to help you but if you don't talk to us, we can't help you," the teary-eyed nurse explained. "Just tell us who did this to you."

I kept having asthma attacks, so they had to keep giving me breathing treatments. And still, I never told.

After I got home from the hospital, I told Bishop Ross about how he made me get into a slip and then beat me.

"He did what?" Bishop Ross asked.

"He made me get in a slip and he beat me."

"Tell him to call me as soon as he gets home. As old as you are, he don't have no business making you get naked and putting you in a slip so he can beat you." Even Bishop Ross didn't understand, making me take off my bra and panties, then put me in a slip to beat me?

Like my grandmother told me, he was mad because I wouldn't fuck him and I also wouldn't stay quiet.

Elder Cooley ended up talking to Bishop Ross about the situation. And of course, I didn't know what was said. But it couldn't have been too much said because the beatings didn't stop. One time Elder Cooley overheard me on the phone with a guy named Keith and he thought I was telling him about how he beat me. So, he rushed into the room and made me get off the phone.

# Chapter 4

# I'm Not Taking It!

**D**uring a night time church service, I was sitting by two of my girlfriends. Elder Cooley tapped one of my friends on her shoulder who was behind me and told her to get my attention. She got my attention, and when I looked over at him, he told me to stop clapping off beat. I was like, *off beat? This is how we clap in church. I don't know nothing else.* Then, right there in church with every seat in the church filled with people, Elder Cooley walked up and slapped me in my face while service was going on. "POW!"

Prior to that, I had been telling my friend Mary about the abuse that was going on. She told me, "The only way he's going to stop beating on you, your mother, and your little brother is when y'all start fighting him back. You gotta start fighting him back to let him know you ain't scared of him. I know you're not scared of him. And his problem is, he knows you're not scared of him."

So, after he slapped me, I started fighting him right in the church. When we started fighting, service had completely stopped. He tried to pick me up and take me outside while I was punching him with all the strength I had in me. At that point, I was tired. I'd had enough and couldn't take it anymore. So, I fought him all the way outside.

When we got home, he tried to chastise me and give me a beating. And we both fought head up like two men in the street. I was throwing stuff at him trying to kill his ass. My mother had to jump between us and beg us to stop. I didn't want to push or hit my mother because I love her. But somebody was about to see that I wasn't going to take that shit anymore and I meant it!

"You better get her!" he yelled while my mother was in the middle of us. "You stupid bitch!" he called me.

"Whatever!" I yelled back at him. "That's what I am, whatever!"

I was talking back and fighting like I had never done before, because I felt like he was out to get me. I no longer cared about him being a Pastor at the Pentecostal Church of God. I had absolutely no respect for him and saw him as just another nigga who was out to get me. He was my enemy at that point. So, while my mother was between us, I looked him in his face and made sure he understood me.

"You want everybody in this house to be scared of you, but I'm not and you know it!" My mother was still between us, then all of a sudden, he just walked away.

"I want her out of my house," he said as he walked away.

"You want me out of your house? Then I'm gone!" But my mother wouldn't let me go anywhere.

I realized that he was no longer trying to chastise me. He was straight up trying to abuse not only me, but my mother and brother also. He beat my mother until she became senseless. She's not even in her right frame of mind to this day.

But that day, he revealed himself to the church again and everybody was saying, "That wasn't necessary. What did she do? She wasn't even doing anything. He just went over and slapped her with all his might!" But did anybody try to help me? Hell no! He hated me and I didn't give a damn because I hated him too. Put two people together who hate each other and you got yourself a war. He started the war, but I was going to end it. And I wasn't going out like a punk either. From that day on, I fought him every time he tried to chastise me. It got to the point where my mother was in the middle of us refereeing.

"I want her out of my house!" was what he said from then on.

"Why you want me out the house? Because I'm standing up for myself and didn't turn out to be a coward or a punk bitch like you tried to make me?"

From then on, every time he approached me with something I didn't like, we just fought it out. Then I started isolating myself and stayed in my room whenever they would go to church events like picnics. They were always going to church members houses to talk and eat, but I never went.

At that point, I really didn't know who I was. All I knew was I became something that I had been raised not to be. I was raised to be respectful to my elders and Pastors, but I had lost that. People told me I was wrong and should've never started fighting Elder Cooley because he was an adult.

"He's a man and you're a little girl. You need to stay in a little girl's place!" And I would've stayed in my place if I was dealing with a real man.

A little while later, Elder Cooley went to see Bishop Ross about the situation that went down between us at church. It was at our next big church meeting when Bishop Ross took his Pastor position away from him.

"If you can't control your own household, then how can you tell the people of God what to do?" Bishop Ross said right in the pulpit, which was true.

I was happy he lost his position. And on our way home from church that Sunday, nobody said anything. The inside of the car was totally silent all the way home. But I was happy, just long as he didn't touch me. And if so, then we were going to go head-to-head. I had been through too much shit at that point. And in-between everything, I ran away from home twice.

One time I ran away with Mary at six o'clock in the morning. I faked like I was going to wait on my school bus. But when Mary came, we hitchhiked us a ride with some middle-aged white guy who drove by.

When we got in his car, he asked us if we wanted something to drink. We were like, "Yeah!" He pulled up at a 7-11. While he was inside, I noticed he had some rolled-up plastic with some blood on it, a rope, and a machete sticking out from under his seat.

"Mary, look at this stuff he got under his back seat."

"What the hell? Bianca, don't touch it! He might be crazy or something. Let's get out of here!"

Instantly, we tried to open our doors to get out. But neither of our doors would open. I tried to pull the lock up, but the lock was gone. That's when we started to panic.

"I can't get out! Mary, open your door!"

"My door won't open either!"

Mary finally decided to crawl out of the driver's door. I hopped over the seat and did the same. We were running down the street when the guy came out of the store yelling, "Hey, where y'all going?" Then he got in his car and started chasing us. "Where y'all going? You little bitches get back here!"

Mary had a friend who lived close by. That's where we ran to. After we explained what happened to the mother of Mary's friend, she just looked at us like we were crazy.

"The two of you need to take y'all asses home!" she told us. "You little heifers, y'all think y'all grown! You can get killed out here. It ain't nothing but the grace of God that kept y'all!"

So, I called Sister Green and told her about it. Sister Green and I were tight at the time. I had spent the night at her house and did her hair on many occasions. She asked me to call her back after a few minutes. When I did, she had called Bishop Ross and told him about my situation. "I called Bishop Ross and he said for you to go home," she told me.

I couldn't believe she called Bishop Ross. What I told her was supposed to be between me and her and I felt like she had betrayed me. But I went home anyway. When I got there my mother was screaming, "Where have you been!" Then my mother gave me a beating, and this was the first chastising I could ever remember my mother giving me.

"I want you to know, I'm not beating you because I want to. It's because Bishop Ross told me to tell you that you're getting beat because he said so, and it's not for running away!" They understood why I ran away, and I guess Bishop Ross opened their eyes to that. "He told me to beat your behind for hitchhiking!"

Not only did he tell her to beat me for hitchhiking, but he also told her to whip me until she got tired. And when Bishop Ross and the other two Bishops of the Pentecostal Church of God say something, the people in the church take it very seriously. So, she literally beat me until she got fucking tired! I was having asthma attacks while she was beating me and everything. I had to take a breathing treatment, then go back and get my ass whipped some more.

She beat me for so long that she had to sit down and drink a can of Coca Cola like she was working or something. I couldn't even accept Bishop Ross for a long time after that because he told my mother to whip me until she got tired. And she took heed and did it like a fool. I think he may have said it as a figure of speech. But for people in our church, when Bishop Ross says something, they do it. If he had said for her to kill me, she probably would've killed me. That's how much they believe in what the man says, and that's crazy.

♫ ♫ ♫ ♫ ♫

One day I guess my mother couldn't take it anymore. That's because she flipped out on me all of a sudden. There were some guys from my high school who came to our house for me. The only reason they came over was so I could tell them where another girl we knew lived. All of the guys looked really thugged out with dreadlocks flying all over the place, gold teeth, and no shirts on. When they knocked on the door, my mother started to flip out.

"Who y'all want?" she asked.

"Is Bianca home?" they asked her.

"Bianca, you got these damn niggas out here in my yard!" she yelled embarrassing me.

"Where Erica stay at?" they asked me when I came to the door.

"She that house right there," I pointed.

My mother was upset because she and Elder Cooley had been fighting. Now for the first time, she took her anger out on me.

"What, you fucking those niggas? You fucking all those niggas?"

"Mama, no I'm not."

"You think you grown?" she yelled just before she charged at me. "What, you wanna hit me? You wanna fight me?'

"Mama no!" I answered while she was in some kind of rage or something.

She charged at me full force like a bull or something, from the living room to my bedroom where I was standing. She had me on my bed then started punching me over and over again in my stomach to the point where I couldn't breathe. Somehow, I managed to push her off of me and she fell to the floor. I got on top of her, held her hands down, then started screaming.

"You think I wanna fight you?"

"Hit me Bianca, hit me! That's what you wanna do! Hit me! That's what you want, you wanna beat on me!"

"Mama no! Mama stop!"

"You wanna fight me? Go ahead hit me!"

"Mama what's wrong with you? I don't wanna fight you! I love you!" Then, I just got up and walked away.

"Bianca I'm sorry," she cried. "I'm sorry Bianca!"

I just threw my hands in the air like, *not you too! You live in this house with me and see what this man do to us and you're about to make me fight you too?* She kept walking through the house following behind me apologizing.

"Bianca wait, wait, wait. Are you mad at me?

"No Mama I'm not mad at you."

"You want some money? Here, take some money."

"No Mama that's okay. I got some money." Then she started pulling out her credit cards. And that's when I knew something was really wrong with her.

Now that I look back on it, I realize it wasn't me who she was doing it to. It was because he had her mind so messed up and what she wanted to do to him, she was doing to me. I guess I was just convenient for her at the time because the stuff she was saying to me didn't make any sense. It was like she couldn't take it anymore and I was the one feeling it. I guess from him beating on her, she felt like that's all everybody wanted to do to her. She took his shit for so many years till that's all she knew.

♫ ♫ ♫ ♫ ♫

Due to all of the violence in my life, I started fighting a lot in high school. I ended up getting kicked out of my high school for hitting my teacher in the face with a board in shop class. Plus, he called me a nigger. After that, I went to the Alternative Learning Center (ALC).

ALC was when regular school didn't work out for you. That was your alternative. It was a school where they sent kids who were on probation or were pregnant. There were extra security and police officers patrolling the premises. The fence around the school was made like a prison fence because we were considered dangerous kids.

ALC was where I met my boyfriend Keith. But at the same time, I was still dating my other boyfriend Garry. Eventually, I found out Keith was dealing drugs. So, I broke up with him. At that age, drugs were like so bad to me and I didn't associate myself with anybody who had anything to do with them. But, before I had broken up with Keith, I showed him how to sneak into our house through a broken window in our bathroom.

I'd sneak him into our house all of the time and we'd be straight up having sex. After I broke up with that fool, I woke up in the middle of the night and he was standing over my bed completely naked. So, I had to sit up there and have sex with him and didn't even want to. And that happened over and over until I got pregnant.

# Chapter 5

## Sean

Not long after I had gotten pregnant, I met a young man at church named Sean. He was from Detroit. We saw each other every six months when our church had its big conventions. In June our church has a convention that lasts for two weeks in Detroit, Michigan. Then, in December we have another convention that lasts for one week in Winter Haven, Florida. So basically, we were raised together seeing each other every six months.

Sean used to send me money when I needed it. Sometimes his whole pay check. He was also the first person who I told I was pregnant. He'd been trying to get me to go out with him since that previous convention before I got pregnant, but I wouldn't.

Whenever we went to the convention, my friends and I would have a bet to see who could get the most phone numbers from all the different out of town guys. And that's what we went to the convention for, to see who could get the most telephone numbers from the different guys throughout the South and Mid-West. Of course, I won the bet. But that's how I started dating Sean.

The tripped-out thing was, I had Sean's number, and I also had his brother Christopher's number. I didn't know they were brothers because they looked like night and day. Christopher is jet black and Sean is yellow looking. With them looking like night and day, how was I supposed to know they were brothers? But I never really liked his brother because whenever we talked, I could sense a really strong gay spirit in him. Sean on the other hand, I really liked him. Good thing a friend of mine pulled me aside one day and let me know what was going on. "What are you doing, don't you know they are brothers?" my friend warned me.

After that, I only talked to Sean. Even though he was really skinny and poor looking, he was really nice to me. His personality was so sweet. Every day he would save me a seat right next to him in service. And even though I didn't want to sit next to him, I did it anyway because I didn't want to diss him. I was really trying to give him a chance. But he was sweating me really hard.

On the last day of the convention in Detroit, we were getting ready to leave when Sean said, "Stand right here and promise not to leave until I come back." I promised, and as soon as he took off around the corner, I took off and got in the car with my mother and Elder Cooley. When Sean saw us driving down the street headed to I 75 South, he ran behind our car trying to stop us.

“Bye Sean!” I opened the door and yelled.” I think that was the meanest thing I had ever done to Sean because he was a really sweet guy.

Back in Florida, I talked to Sean off and on and I was really starting to dig him. He was aware that I had a lot of guys who liked me. And, he was also aware of my baby daddy Keith. I remember when I told him I was pregnant. It was during the church convention in December. Sean was sharing a room with his friends at the Howard Johnson Hotel. That’s where we stood in the hallway and talked about our relationship.

“Why Bianca, why won’t you be my girl?” he asked me. He sounded so funny to me because people from the Mid-West tend to sound really proper. They just don’t have that country slang like us country folks.

“I can’t Sean.”

“Why not?”

“Look at my stomach,” then he put his hand on my stomach.

“Oh my God,” he said with his mouth wide open.

“I’m pregnant, well at least I think I’m pregnant. I almost know I’m pregnant.”

“I don’t care. I’m in love with you,” he told me with both of his hands still on my stomach.

“But Sean, I’m pregnant.”

"I don't care. Are you hungry or anything?"

Little stuff like that made me fall in love with him. I was like, *damn, this guy is feeling my stomach and I'm telling him I'm pregnant and he doesn't even care.*

Sean's friends left out of the room so we could be alone. Me and Sean went in and started kissing each other. He always had a hard on for some reason. And I was always horny as well. But I could've waited. But we both got naked anyway, laid on the bed, then he put a condom on. He touched my breast and told me I was so beautiful. Then he rubbed my hips with both of his hands.

"Man, do you know how fine you are?"

I had no idea how sexy I was. At that point, I was still shy. But not too shy to take control of the situation. That's when I got ready to sit on him and he pushed me off of him.

"This ain't right," he told me.

"Do you want me to lay on my back?"

"Yeah, lay on your back."

I laid on my back, then he started kissing my breast. I was nervous because it was our first time together. And I got to admit, Sean had the biggest dick I had seen at that point in my life. I was like, *oh my God* when I saw the condom with his dick in it coming at me. I thought to myself, *what the fuck? He's gonna bust my pussy open!* But I was feeling really freaky right about then and decided to do him anyway.

Every time he got ready to put it in, he would stop. So, I got confused.

"What's wrong?" I asked him.

"Nothing," he answered while still hard. Then he did the same thing again.

"Sean what's wrong?"

"Bianca I can't do this."

"Why not?"

"Because you're too good for this."

"What?"

"You're too good for this and I can't mess over you like this."

"Mess over me? What do you mean?"

I was dripping wet and could smell my pussy and perspiration. So, it was time to fuck. In my mind I was saying, *now you wanna tell me this? I ain't no good? Fuck me please!* I wanted it so bad and I don't think I've ever wanted to have sex with a man that bad. But what he told me really offended me. My self-esteem was already low and I felt like the ugliest person in the world. I thought I was too skinny and my hips were too big. I had been taken advantage of, abused and molested, Therefore, what little bit of self-esteem I had left, he took it.

"How the hell can you get me naked in the bed then resist me?"

"It's only because I love you." After that, we put our clothes back on. "Are you okay?"

"Yeah, I'm okay."

"Are you sure?"

"Yeah, I'm fine."

I left the room. While walking down the hallway, I saw my friend Roy McDougal. So, I stopped him to get his take on the situation.

"Roy, you're a man, tell me what you think about this. Sean just had me in the room and we were naked. He put a condom on, the mood was right. He was rubbing and kissing my body. His dick was on hard and everything. But then he stopped. In the middle of everything, he just stopped and told me I was too good for that."

I stood there looking at Roy, then burst out crying.

"Tell me, am I unattractive or something? Am I that ugly? What did I do wrong?"

"Sean really loves you Bianca and everybody can see it. He respects you and cares about you."

The next day, Sean and I talked about what happened in-between church services. Back at the hotel, I was walking up the stairs in my green and white wrap around skirt as Sean walked behind me holding my hips.

"Your body is like an hour glass," he said when we sat at the top of the stairs. Then he mumbled something.

"What did you say Sean?"

"Nothing," he answered as I stood up to re-wrap my skirt.

"Lord just one more time, just one more time," he mumbled again. And that time I heard him.

"What do you mean just one more time?"

"If I get one more time," he started beating himself up with regret, "I can't believe I didn't. I'm sorry, but this time I'm ready. I'm going all the way through with it."

We went back into his hotel room to try it again. And all I have to say is **MY LORD, MY LORD, MY LORD!** God smiled on us that day. The sex was good. I wasn't faking my moans or anything because he was really making me moan from deep down inside of me. He gave me the best sex I had ever had.

Sean stood tight by my side that whole convention and we developed a strong bond. From then on, our six months apart seemed like six years. When he went home, he started sending me money for my maternity clothes and anything else I needed for the baby. He was supporting my child when he wasn't even born yet. But the funny thing about this situation was not only was I pregnant, but my mother was pregnant also. My mother and I were straight up pregnant at the same time *(you know you ghetto when)* and for the first time in my life, I felt sorry for Elder Cooley. He was living in a house with two pregnant women.

After I started showing and everybody in the church found out I was pregnant, I got put out of the church. They disfellowship people when they commit a sin like having sex and getting pregnant. This was forbidden and Bishop Ross would stand in the pulpit and announce in front of everybody that you were put out. You could still go to the church and participate, but you were not considered an active member and God looked down on you for what you did.

So being put out of the church was devastating. To us, it was the worst thing that could happen in the world. So, I clung tight to my mother and we got along together like peanut butter and jelly. We'd both be in the same bed with our bellies touching and craving Reese's Pieces. I had my son *Little Keith* first. Then two months later, my mother had her daughter, my little sister, and my son's aunt. I went back to church regularly. When they had a "Coming Home" line, I got in it and begged the Lord for forgiveness. After I stood in front of the entire church and told the Lord I was sorry, he then forgave me and I was back in the church.

♫ ♫ ♫ ♫ ♫

My son and my little sister were raised together. And for a long time, people thought they were twins. We'd stroll them around in double strollers and sometimes dress them alike. Little fights still broke out around the house. But it seemed like once those babies got there, some tension was broken. It was new life and a new beginning. Well, at least that's how I felt. I guess my parents figured, *there's nothing else we can do, she already gotten herself pregnant and had a baby.* Maybe that's what they were trying to prevent. So, they kind of laid off of me after that.

Sean and I still only saw each other every six months. But we talked over the phone a lot. And it was over the phone when he asked me to marry him. He FedExed me a heart shaped engagement ring with some fake diamonds around the top of it. I was swept off my feet when I got the ring. Therefore, the next church convention in Detroit, I made sure I had my own hotel room.

I rode to Detroit with my mother and Elder Cooley. Soon as we got there, I gave my son to my aunt to care for him while I planned to have myself a ball. And a ball I had. But three days after we arrived in Detroit, my mother and Elder Cooley just upped and went back to Florida, leaving me stranded in Detroit.

Before I realized they had left me, they were arguing and fighting about the house we lived in back in Florida. I guess they were being evicted and had to hurry up and get back home or something. A lot of times we would use all of our money to go to our church convention, even though we couldn't afford it. But our Bishop always told us, "The Lord will provide a way."

Someone told me the reason they left me was because I thought I was grown, so they were going to treat me like I was grown. Whatever the case was, the fact is, they left me stranded in Detroit, Michigan and went back to Fort Meyers, Florida. That's the kind of shit I had to deal with. How are they going to leave a child in another state like that? They took all the other kids, but left me. I had no money or food, and thank God for Sean because he really took care of me. He fed me breakfast, lunch and dinner every single day and even gave me some money.

I stayed in Detroit for the rest of the convention then caught a ride back with my aunt who lived in Jacksonville, Florida. About a month after I was back in Fort Meyers, I found out I was pregnant by Sean. Nine months later, I had our daughter Tina. And then I got put out of the church again.

After I had Tina, Elder Cooley started making a big deal about me and my kids living in his house.

"I pay the bills here! I bring the food in here!" were some of the things he made a big deal about. As usual, he tried to make me feel like I wasn't shit. And as far as he was concerned, I wasn't going to be nothing but shit, if that.

One day my mother was telling her kids what to eat before she went to work.

"Y'all can get some cereal, but don't eat up those babies WIC cereal because they gotta eat to. Y'all can go to school and eat there if it's not enough." I told my little brother Derrick not to eat that box of Cheerios because I bought that with my WIC check.

"And next time don't go and eat up all the cereal in the house, then turn around and eat my baby's cereal! Mama already told y'all not to do that!" As I was talking to Derrick, Elder Cooley flipped out on me.

"This is my house! You don't tell nobody what to eat in here! I don't care if you did bring it in here! You don't pay a damn dime on nothing in here! You ain't nothing but a hoe!"

"Whatever," I smartly replied, "whatever!"

"I want you out of my house you damn hoe! Get out of my house!"

"You ain't said nothing," I told him then went and started packing me and my kids bags. Right after that, I left.

I went down the street to a friend's house and explained what happened to her and her mother. After I finished explaining, their response was, "What? That's a damn shame. He's been wanting to put you out ever since day one! You can stay here for as long as you need to get yourself together."

I bounced from house to house for a while until finally I ended up in Jacksonville, Florida with my Aunt Donna. Sean came to Jacksonville to be with me and our child. And we all stayed at Aunt Donna's house together. We planned to get married and start a new life in Florida. So, Sean started looking for work. Three months later, Sean still had no work. That's when he realized Florida wasn't where he wanted his home to be. He became sad and depressed and told me he missed his family back home. After three months, Sean went back to Detroit.

I ended up leaving Florida and went to Detroit to start a life with Sean and the kids. My kids and I stayed with a friend of mine from our church name Ann Gordon. Ann was living with her mother at the time, and her mother gladly welcomed me and my kids. Sean was still out of work but he said he had something lined up. Plus, somebody from the church was going to let us rent one of their homes.

Not long after I arrived in Detroit, Sean took me to church. He made an appointment for us to talk to the head Bishop there named Bishop Duren. Inside Bishop Duren's office, Sean told him he wanted to marry me.

"So y'all trying to be in love?" Bishop Duren asked.

“Yes Sir,” we both answered.

“That’s good. That’s the way the Lord wants it,” he said nodding his head.

Bishop Duren gave us his blessing and permitted us to get married. I was so happy when we left his office because I felt like Sean had just rescued me from a horrible life. He was my knight in shining armor.

# Chapter 6

# Exhale

I went back to Florida to tell my mother how Bishop Duren had given us permission to get married. Plus, to get the rest of my belongings. The day before I was to leave Florida for the last time, I got a call from Sean's sister-in-law Yolanda, who was also a member of our church.

"Every time I see Sean, I also see Ann Gordon. Are you two still together, because I just want to know?"

"Yes, me and Sean are still together."

"Are you sure? Because every time I see him, he's with her. She rides in the front seat of his car and they be off into their own little world in the back of the church. Sunday at church, I was coming out of the kitchen and they were on the stairway talking. I'm not trying to start nothing, but I just thought you should know."

After that, I called Sean and asked him about it.

"Sean, be honest with me and tell me what's going on. Is there somebody else? If you don't want to be with me, then you need to let me know. Let's not make a mistake that we'll both regret."

"What are you talking about?" he asked me.

"I heard you're messing around with Ann."

"Me and Ann been friends for years. It's nothing."

"Okay, well if you don't want to be honest with me, then I'm going to call Ann and ask her myself."

I called Ann to see if she was going to say something about it. But she didn't. I talked to Sean about it again and he demanded that I tell him where I had heard the rumor."

"Who told you this because somebody's hating on me and don't want to see us together?" I told him it wasn't important who told me. Then I let the situation go. But right after that, I got a call from Ann and she was confessing.

"I'm sorry about what's going on," she told me. "But Sean needs to be the one to tell you what happened."

"What happened," I asked while pissed off.

She didn't say what happened and told me I needed to talk to Sean. But fuck Sean! I just had that man's baby, my parents were flipping out on me because of it. Plus, I thought I had a future with him. As for Ann, that slimy bitch! We were supposed to be really tight. But all along she was trying to take my man. I guess all the years we've been friends didn't mean nothing to her. So, I called Sean back.

"She already called me and told me what was going on. I just want you to confirm it and tell me the truth. Don't lie to me!" He came out and told me they just kissed and that was that. "Do you want to be with her?" I asked him. "If you want to be with her, just tell me and I won't even come back to Detroit. I'll let it be what it is."

"No Bianca, I don't want to be with her. I love you. I'm sorry and this should've never happened."

I was so upset about what happened, I had to call Bishop Ross and talk to him about it. After I told him what happened, he said everybody makes mistakes and we need to learn to forgive people. Then we came to the conclusion that it was only a kiss. I forgave Sean and went back to Detroit.

I was so happy to be there and we were in love all over again. We stayed with Yolanda and Sean's brother until we were able to move into our own house. Yolanda was a real cool chick. A lot of people tried to poison me by telling me how she was a snake. But she made us feel very welcome in their home.

I saw snow for the very first time in my life while in Detroit. Sean and I were coming out of a CVS store. I was trying to hurry back to the car because it was cold. As Sean was placing the kids in the car and talking to me at the same time. Then I felt something wet hit my nose. I thought he had accidentally spit on me. But then it happened again and he wasn't even facing me.

"Something just fell on me," I told Sean.

"That's snow baby," he came over and hugged me. "This is your first snow."

"Oh my God. I thought you were spitting on me," I laughed.

Whenever it would snow, I would take my kids outside and we'd make snow angels in the front yard. To me, the snow was the most beautiful thing I had ever seen.

After two weeks, we moved into a house on the Westside of Detroit. The street was called Northlawn and we rented the house from a member of our church. We weren't married yet and us living together with my two kids was a big problem for Sean's family and a lot of church members. A lot of self-righteous people were saying we were just shacking up and shouldn't be living like that.

But I loved our new home. It was a big house with two bedrooms on the first floor, three bedrooms upstairs and a basement. We didn't have much when we started out because Sean didn't have a job. But he eventually landed a job at a restaurant. We saved up enough money to upgrade his beat-up car to a slightly better car and we were doing okay. We were happy about having our own place and new wheels. But we were still poor.

We had an old TV that was sitting in a chair and no furniture. But it didn't matter because we had each other. It wasn't long before Sean hooked up with some people who gave us some furniture and that was a blessing in itself. They gave us a queen size bed, a car bed for my son Little Keith, and a baby crib for our daughter Tina.

Everything was perfect. No arguing or fighting. After a while, Sean landed a better job at a factory. So, I had to adjust to staying in that big house while he worked longer hours. But I was still happy. I was like, *wow, I got my own life here. I don't have nobody trying to beat on me and I don't have to live in a domestic violent environment.* I was finally able to exhale… at least that's what I thought.

# Chapter 7

# I'm Married Now

**O**ne evening Sean came in from work and soon as he hit the door, he had his pants halfway down. And instantly, we were kissing and moaning, "Ummm, yes baby!" That's how we were with each other. Just two passionate love making people. We loved to make love to each other and we were having sex like crazy all over the house. Soon as he'd walk in the door, the kids would be asleep, dinner would be on the table and he wouldn't even be out of his work clothes good before we would go at it.

We made it to the bedroom where he laid me on the bed. I was completely naked and playing with myself. Sean took his pants off, unbuttoned his shirt and laid on top of me. We were kissing, moaning, licking and squeezing on each other. And then the phone rang. Sean stopped kissing me then reached over and answered. "Hello. Who is this?" he asked the caller as I rubbed my feet on his dick. "Oh, praise the Lord Bishop Duren!"

Sean quickly started putting his pants back on like Bishop Duren had straight up walked into his own room and caught us fucking in his bed. He zipped his pants up while looking scared to death of what we were about to do. I just looked at him like, *Bishop Duren can't see you!* He was actually so scared that he tucked his work shirt back into his pants. It's crazy as hell how those men *(the Bishops)* have that kind of power over people.

Bishop Duren called and asked Sean when were we getting married?

"Soon Bishop," Sean explained. "We already went downtown to see about getting the marriage license. And now it won't be long."

Bishop Duren told Sean he understood. But we needed to hurry up and do what we needed to do. Right then, I knew people were in our business and telling it back to Bishop Duren. One of the people who I knew was in our business was Sean's grandmother. She didn't like me and didn't want Sean to be with me. Plus, by me being put out of the church, a lot of people felt like no one should deal with me until I got back in.

A week later, we got married. And I guess since I was married, I was officially back in the church and an active member of the Pentecostal Church of God.

It was a cold snowy day in February when we had our very small wedding at the church. I really didn't want to have a wedding ceremony. Instead, I wanted to simply go into Bishop Duren's office and let him marry us. But we had a ceremony anyway because two of Sean's brothers talked him into it.

It was a normal wedding, but I had no family support. Not one single person from my family was there. Not even my own mother. And only three of Sean's family members came to support us *(Yolanda, her husband and Christopher).* Christopher even got on the organ and played "Here Comes the Bride." Our pastor Elder Strong married us and there were an additional five church members who came to our wedding to show us some support.

A lot of Sean's family members claimed he didn't tell them about the wedding. But Sean said he did tell them. I guess our wedding wasn't a big enough deal to his family. But I wasn't surprised one bit because they acted as if they never liked me anyway. For some reason, they thought I was some type of whore and Sean was making a big mistake by marrying me.

We got married anyway, and was happy with our small ceremony. And even though we were the newlyweds, Sean and I treated the few people at our wedding out to the Olive Garden restaurant.

An elderly couple at the Olive Garden sent a waitress to our table to ask Sean a question. "The gentleman sitting over there wants to know if it would be okay if he bought your table a bottle of champagne. He said your wife is the most beautiful bride he's seen in a long time."

It was a nice compliment from the strange old man. When the bottle was brought over to us, he and his wife both started clapping their hands for us. Then as they were leaving, they came over and kissed me on my cheek.

"You look like a princess, you're so beautiful," the wife told me.

When Sean and I got home, we made a pallet on the living room floor. We had our empty champagne bottle that we brought home from the restaurant. We also had two bottles of wine we picked up from the store, some cake, and a few other desserts we brought home from the restaurant. Our night was magical, and the most romantic night I had ever had.

Then, two days later I heard a knock on the door while I was in the bathroom. I rushed to the door as fast as I could, only to find Ann getting back into her car and driving off. *What was she doing over here,* I wondered? I called Ann later on that evening to see what she wanted. She told me she wanted to tell me face-to-face how she was sorry about what had happened between her and Sean. She said she felt like she owed me an apology.

"What are you talking about Ann?" I asked. "He told me the only thing that happened was a kiss."

"Is that what he told you?" she asked me.

"Yes!"

"Oh. Is that really all he told you?"

"Ann, did something else happen?"

I was getting angry because the situation was starting to hit me hard. We were only married for two days and still had the champagne and wine bottles laying around. And now Ann is telling me some mess about her and Sean.

"Ann, you know that's fucked up! You're supposed to be my friend! And you got the nerves to come over two days after we got married to bring this shit up! Why didn't you tell me about this before we got married? This is some fucked up shit!"

I was in a rage because in so many words, she told me she had fucked Sean. So later on, when Sean walked in the house, I fussed at him about it. Then we got into a big argument over it. I had my finger all in his face telling him how he wasn't shit. And then he shoved me into the stairs. I fell on the stairs, then got up and pushed him back. Then, we started straight up fighting.

As we were fighting, Sean picked up the champagne bottle the old man bought us and he busted it across my head. I fell to the floor, feeling like I was about to pass out. I gained my composure and slowly got off the floor. Then some blood rolled down my face, and that's when I realized my forehead was busted open.

There I was again, feeling like shit while thinking to myself, *damn, I got put out of my mother's house, I've left Florida, and now I'm in a house where I have to fight my own husband. I can't win for losing. What kind of fucked up life is this?* I walked away from Sean and gathered up my kids. I put them in the double stroller and we started walking down the snow-covered streets.

Before I left the house, I called Yolanda and told her I would be walking down 7 Mile Road and to come pick me up because Sean and I had gotten into it. And as cold as it was outside, I was walking down the street with my kids while holding a towel with some ice in it on my forehead. There was a big knot on my forehead that was getting larger by the minute.

When Yolanda pulled up, she parked alongside of the road, then got out to help us in.

"What the hell happened to you?" she asked looking at the big knot on my forehead. "Hell naw! Sean needs his ass kicked!"

"Yolanda don't tell nobody about this," I pleaded. "Just take me to your house."

Sean ended up calling Yolanda's phone to apologize to me. He told me he was trying to hit the bottle against the wall. And for some reason, I believed him. So, me and the kids went back home.

Even though I went back home to Sean, I was still homesick and wanted to go back to Florida. But I couldn't go back because Elder Cooley had put me out. I didn't even feel like I could call my mother and tell her about what I had gone through only two days after my wedding. That's when I started feeling like I didn't have anybody.

♫ ♫ ♫ ♫ ♫

They say if you grow up in a domestic violent home, eventually you will have one of your own. And that's what happened to me.

♫ ♫ ♫ ♫ ♫

# Chapter 8

# People Don't Like Me

**O**ur life went on, but the situation between Ann and Sean was still a hard pill for me to swallow. I had given up my life for that man. I had scholarship offers concerning my music career. I gave it up to get married because I thought he loved me. But now, all we do is argue about this Ann.

Eventually, the situation died down. But then, my health was starting to give me problems. Yolanda took me to a clinic where two doctors practiced. One of them was a man name Dr. Everett Hamrick. Dr. Hamrick was a tall man of African descent. He had a head full of what we called "good hair." He ended up being my primary care physician and I desperately needed him because I had chronic asthma, upper respiratory disease and was having acute asthma attacks.

He took my blood and did a pap smear. Everything came back negative with no STDs. He prescribed me some pills to help me with my breathing, and I was on my way.

Three months later, I went back to Dr. Hamrick because I was nauseous, fatigue, had stomach and lower back pain, could barely breathe, plus I had a fever of 103. Come to find out, I was coming down with the flu. Dr. Hamrick asked me a question in a low voice.

"Who's the lucky fellow?"

"What do you mean who's the lucky fellow?" I asked confusingly.

"You can tell me, I'm your doctor. I'm not going to tell anybody. Who are you cheating with? I remember you told me you just got married and the two of you are cheating already?"

"Dr. Hamrick I'm not cheating on my husband. What are you talking about?"

"Well, you have a small case of chlamydia."

"Wait a minute! What do you mean I have a small case of chlamydia?"

"I know you have to be cheating because when I did your blood work and pap smear three months ago everything was negative. If you're being honest with me, I'd hate to be the one to tell you, but your husband is cheating on you."

I was hurt by what he told me. At the time, things were going kind of good between me and Sean. I didn't want any more arguing or fighting between us. Therefore, I didn't say anything to Sean about it. I came on him in a different way.

"Sean, will you be honest with me because I want to ask you something?" I asked him while we were lying in bed. "It's not about you and Ann. But honey, are you cheating on me?"

"No," he answered really quickly. "No Bianca."

"Sean, are you sure?"

"Yes I'm sure, I promise."

I knew he was lying to me. But I didn't want any more fighting. Plus, everything was fine between us. So, I told him Dr. Hamrick said I had strep throat and it was contagious. Therefore, I needed him to take some antibiotics with me because it wasn't going to help if only I took them and he infected me again.

Sean believed me and that's how I got him to take the antibiotics. Later on, I went back to my doctor and my STD was gone. But being married was really stressing me out. We were newlyweds and already on our second infidelity. I was living in a big city and didn't know many people. Therefore, I felt all alone because I didn't have any family members who I could call on for help. My mother was totally clueless to what was going on, and when she did call me, I faked it. "Yeah Mama, everything's okay. The kids are doing fine and we're happy together."

I'm a very private person. Plus, I felt like if I told her, she and Elder Cooley would've probably been happy and said, "That's what you get for leaving! You should've stayed in Florida!" But either way, I would've been going through the same domestic violence bullshit.

♫ ♫ ♫ ♫ ♫

I spent most of my time in church, going to the hospital for my asthma, and going to see Dr. Hamrick. My asthma kept me really sick because there's a big difference between the weather in Florida and Detroit. My asthma was acting up so bad to where I was going to the hospital almost every three days. The same paramedics would come pick me up almost every time, and they knew me by my first name. I went to DMC Sinai Grace Hospital so much that the doctors even knew me by name.

I was under a lot of stress due to my health and Sean cheating on me. Whenever he left the house, I feared he was going to cheat. Even with that, I still wanted our marriage to work and I prayed to the Lord about the situation. I felt like I didn't have anybody else, so the Lord was where my help was coming from.

I would go to church on Tuesday evening and Friday evening. On Sundays, I would be at church mostly all day. I would go to Sunday morning Bible School, Sunday noon service, Sunday YPU service, then Sunday evening service. If there was a special prayer or meeting in between those services, best believe I was there as well because I really wanted my marriage to work. I loved that man and wanted him to love me too.

Because of Ann and him giving me a STD, I felt like he didn't love me. But he eventually came out and told me the truth about him and Ann.

"Why didn't you tell me the truth when I was in Florida?" I asked Sean.

"I lied because I was afraid you wouldn't marry me."

"What right do you have to do that? You basically made the decision for me by lying to me."

If he would've told me the truth at first, I would have stayed home. I would've never walked into something like this with my eyes wide open.

Therefore, the only way I knew to help us was to get more involved in church. I even sang in the choir, thinking it was somehow going to help us. But then our marriage started to go even more downhill.

♫ ♫ ♫ ♫ ♫

It was summer time and our church convention had just ended. Sean had been spending a lot of time with his old girlfriend from our church named Dawn Davison. Dawn had moved down South a couple of years ago. But she stayed in Detroit after the convention to spend some time with her family. One day I was walking through the house and I saw Sean on the phone. When he saw me, he quickly got off the phone and walked away so fast you could say he was running.

"Sean, who were you talking to?" I asked, fearing he was cheating on me.

"I was talking to Dawn," he answered embarrassedly.

"Why you sneaking and talking to her? What's going on? Are you fucking her too?"

"I just wanted to call her and spend some time with her while she was in town."

"Okay, do you want me spending time with my ex? How would you feel if I called Garry and asked him do he want to hook up?"

Dawn and her family were some of the people who caused a lot of problems in our marriage. Basically, it was her mother and some of the people they hung around. As far as going to church, Dawn's mother made it real hard for me because she stayed in our business. We were supposed to be the "people of God" and they were behaving more like the people of the Devil.

One Sunday after service, Dawn's mother was sitting in the basement. Sean and I were headed to our car while I had Tina in my arm and Little Keith by his hand. As we walked past Dawn's mother, she stopped Sean. I also stopped because Sean tapped me.

"No, I don't want her, I just want to talk to you," she burst out and told Sean.

"Stay right there Bianca," was what he told me.

"We're having a dinner at our house and I want you to know you're invited, and just you only," she told Sean.

How rude and disrespectful she was. And that's just the kind of treatment I got from people at the Detroit church. I was standing right there when she said it. So, I threw my hand up like *whatever,* then walked away with my kids.

"Bianca, Bianca," Sean pleaded as I walked away. It was like every time I went to church, there was something new with that Davison family. I think it was all because Dawn didn't like me because she felt like I broke up their little fling or whatever they had going on. But they gave me a lot of hell and that hurt me.

Looking back, I have to ask myself, "Why would I let that affect me?" I was so into church and I thought the people there were supposed to be kind and loving. Dawn's mother was over fifty years old and I couldn't understand why she would be acting so childish, especially towards young people.

It began to be too stressful for me to go to church. They would always do something to hurt my feelings. They were just a bunch of females who were jealous of me and I had to deal with it, at church out of all places. Then one day

Sean called Dawn and she called him back. I answered the phone and felt so humiliated after I hung up on her. The situation bothered me so much till Sean and I had to go and talk to Bishop Duren about it… for the second time.

"Sean and I have been in here before and talked to you about these same people," I explained to Bishop as I told him what the Davison family were doing. "Every time we come to church, they'll speak to him and won't even look at me. Then, they will hug and kiss all on him and won't have nothing to say to me."

"If they can't speak to your wife, then you don't speak to them," Bishop Duren told Sean.

They were making it so hard for me to be a new member of the Pentecostal Church of God in Detroit. Sean eventually apologized to me in Bishop Duren's office for the hell he was making in our home.

"How would you feel if a man came up to me and hugged and kissed all over me and didn't say anything to you?" I asked Sean. But most of the time, men don't even do stupid shit like that. It was a female thing I was dealing with. And even after I expressed myself and Bishop Duren said what he said in the office, nothing changed. After that, we started to fight and got physical about the situation.

One Sunday we had a fight because I walked up and saw Ann and Sean hugging and talking after church. Soon as I walked up, she walked away and didn't say anything to me.

"I'm your wife and I feel so disrespected," I yelled at Sean. "Especially when this is the same bitch that caused us so many problems!" When we got home, we started fighting. It seemed like every time we went to church, we came home and fought about another woman, or the Davison family.

One day, Dawn's younger sister Tiffany was outside the church having a conversation with Sean. When I walked up, she just walked away.

"Don't be like that," Sean told Tiffany.

"Let her be how she wanna be!" I yelled. "I'm going to the car!"

"Bianca, Bianca, don't go nowhere!" He was talking to me so rudely it seemed like he was trying to embarrass me in front of her. So, we argued about it all the way home.

At the house, we physically fought about it, and this was one time when he straight up started choking the shit out of me. After he finished choking me, he put a blue laundry basket over my head. He started jerking it back and forth with my head in it and held me down with his knee in my back the whole time.

After the fight, he went in one room and I went into another. We eventually ended up in the same bed before the night was over. The next morning, he went to work as usual. I had bruises all over me from the fight. Now, I was getting used to seeing them. When Sean came home from work, he apologized and told me our fighting had to stop. I agreed and we promised not to fight each other anymore.

Not long after the phone situation between Sean and Dawn, I went to church and people were laughing in my face and talking about me like a dog. They would sit right behind me and say, "She's the stupid one. He was just fooling around with Ann and now he's trying to mess around with me."

I talked to Dawn face to face. When I went to see her at her sisters' house, all five of her sisters were standing on the porch staring at me.

"Dawn, can I talk to you?" I asked standing in the walkway. She came off the porch and seemed to be taking me as a joke.

"Wasn't he just fucking Ann?" She asked me. "And now he's trying to fuck me too!"

"I don't have a problem with you Dawn. My problem is with him. All I want to know is the truth."

"I don't have a problem with you either, but you need to check your man. That nigga is on me. I'm not thinking about him. All he wants is some pussy."

I stood there and cried my eyes out in front of her and it was all a big joke to her. Later I felt like a fool for standing there and letting her see me cry for what she helped do to my marriage. I should've never gone to her in the first place. At church, we were told not to hate your brother or sister. And if you do, then you go to them and you work it out. That's how I was raised and I didn't want any problems with anybody. However, that family is not the type of people who you can talk to because they live for drama and confusion. Misery loves company and they are miserable and want everybody else to be miserable with them.

That night Sean and I were up all night arguing about Dawn. When morning came and it was time for him to go to work, we were still arguing. He got in the car and as he was backing out of the driveway, I ran to the car and hit the windshield with my hand. The windshield cracked when I hit it because that's just how mad I was. I felt like I was getting beat up because of some dumb shit he was doing with the people at church. So, I ended up calling Bishop Duren at his office.

"Bishop, I don't think I'll ever be the same again," in tears I cried on the phone. "These people are causing so much confusion in my home. I'm getting my head bust and bruises all over my body from fighting."

"All of this fighting is happening more and more often," Bishop explained. "They try to say that everybody is doing it. But everybody is not doing it! I'm not doing it and Bishop Ross is not doing it! This is a shame!"

"Bishop I don't want the marriage anymore. I give up. I want to go home."

"I know it's rough, but I believe you are stronger than that and you'll pull through everything."

The Bishop encouraged me to stay strong. But after I got off the phone, I still wanted to go home. I was feeling really out of place. My support was supposed to be the church, but the people at the church were making it harder for me.

After the phone conversation, I started having an asthma attack. I arrived at Dr. Hamrick's and he told me I needed to be put on oxygen because my oxygen level was way too low. I was light headed and my toes and fingers were tingling. There wasn't enough oxygen getting to my brain. He ordered me some oxygen, and the next day it arrived at my house.

Dr. Hamrick also prescribed me a lot of medication and some of it was narcotics. He told me the narcotics would help me relax and sleep better. I was on a sleeping pill called Restoril, a pill called Paxil for depression, Benadryl 50mg, Tylenol #3, and another pill I could never figure out how to pronounce. The medications were making me sleep a lot. But even though I slept a lot, the arguing between me and Sean had gotten worse.

Then I noticed how I was doing less around the house and giving less care to my kids. I wasn't cleaning up or cooking. All I wanted to do was sleep.

After a while, I tried to stop taking the medications because we wanted to have another baby for some strange reason. Even though our marriage was bad, we were still trying to get through it. He started to see some of the things people were doing to us. And after that, he was teaming up with me to make me feel like we were in this thing together. But I was still being deceived because not long after that, I found out Sean was messing around with one of Bishop Duren's granddaughters named Crystal Duren.

I got on our computer and read some emails they had been sending each other. They had been writing love letters to each other and had an affair going on for God knows how long. It was like before I could get over one woman, he had another one. I couldn't even heal from one situation before he put us in another one.

Again, he apologized and promised never to do it again. Then he started going to counseling with Bishop Duren about his cheating, arguing and fighting. Sometimes I went to counseling with Sean. In counseling, Bishop Duren told us to stay prayerful and to keep coming to church.

I can't say that Sean was a straight monster because we both were young and foolish. Two young people entering into a marriage can be really stressful. So, we tried to work on our problems by talking to each other in order to get to know each other a little better.

Sean was given an active position in the Sunday YPU services for the Young People Department at church. One thing that was weighing heavy on me was the fact that the same bitch, Crystal Duren worked in the YPU service. And to make things worse, they worked side by side with each other. I told Bishop Duren about this at counseling. And once again, he told me, "I believe you are stronger than that. I believe you can take it."

I accepted what the Bishop told me. But it was still hard for me to go to church. Everybody there was already saying, "She's stupid for staying with him. Sean really doesn't want to be with her. He only married her because she got pregnant and had his baby."

But still I was trying to be that church going woman they raised me up to be. Basically, I was trying to be what everybody was telling me I was supposed to be. "A child of God would be this way," they would tell me. "Fight the good fight of faith and hold on," and I was trying to do that. "Press on. Strive on," so that's what I was doing.

The church is why I was married. I wasn't married because I wanted to be. I was married because Bishop Duren was encouraging me to stay in the marriage and work it out. So, I stayed. Then I got pregnant again. When I got pregnant, things calmed down and I felt like all of our problems were resolved. We didn't fight and we didn't even do too much arguing at that time.

# Chapter 9

# Davenport

Towards the end of my pregnancy the doctor told me my placenta was attached to my cervix. This was detrimental because it was supposed to be attached to my stomach wall. And with that, I was expected to die while giving birth.

The doctor and some specialists told me and Sean how I needed an emergency c-section and I was not going to live through the birth. The baby was to go home with Sean and he had to care for it because I was not going to live. That was the worst news two expecting parents could ever hear. We both sat there devastated.

The doctor explained, "After I cut your stomach open and we remove the baby, then I have to remove the placenta. A c-section is already a high-risk procedure, and that's even before removing the placenta from your cervix. It can't stay in there for long. And soon as we remove the placenta, that's when the problem will begin. You will start to hemorrhage, and then you'll bleed to death."

They scheduled me for an emergency c-section and the date was only two weeks away. I'll never forget that date because that's the day they told me I was going to die. I broke down in the doctor's office while wondering who was going to take care of my kids.

"I know you are church people," the doctor told us. "You need to call your church and have them pray for your situation."

Walking out of the doctor's office, I felt numb. I had never been that scared in my entire life. But little did I know was, the Lord had something better planned for me. When the date came, the doctor and hospital staff prepared me for surgery. Then right there in front of all of us, a miracle was performed. While the nurse was doing the ultrasound to see where they were going to cut me, she kept repositioning the camera.

"It's been moved," the nurse told us.

"Thank you Jesus, thank you Jesus!" Sean and I both yelled out."

They didn't believe my placenta had been moved. They rolled my bed over to a bigger ultrasound machine. And there, they discovered the same thing. The placenta had been moved. Then, they took all of the equipment off of me and sent me home.

I did not have to have an emergency c-section like they planned. I felt like my life was spared. God heard my cry. The Lord had something different planned and I was so thankful for that. Sean and I both prayed to the Lord and He answered our prayer. He allowed the placenta to move over to the right just enough so I could have a vaginal labor. Not long after that, I gave birth to our beautiful daughter Faith.

♫ ♫ ♫ ♫ ♫

One day I had to help Sean and his sister get some FIA assistance for their mother. I wasn't even supposed to be out of the house because I had not too long ago given birth. But they acted as if they didn't know anything about the FIA system. So, because I was nice, I went with them.

At the FIA office Sean, his sister and their mother went into the social worker's office while I sat in the lobby with my kids. They were back there for a long time. Then the social worker came out without them. She walked over to me and started talking to my kids and rubbing them on their heads. I thought she was just the average social worker at the time who was just being nice to my kids.

One night about two months after we went to the FIA office, Sean and I were getting ready to have sex. When Sean took off his clothes, he had dried up pussy cum all over his dick and between his legs. I was hurt out of this world and just went nuts.

"What the fuck is this?" I asked, knowing it wasn't from me because we hadn't had sex in three days. I screamed and yelled at him, then went into the bathroom and slammed the door. "Why are you doing this to me? Sean who is it, who is it?"

Later on, Sean ended up confessing how he had been seeing a woman named Antoinette Davenport. And she just so happened to be the same woman that was working at the FIA office.

"Who is Antoinette," I asked Sean.

"Antoinette Davenport," he answered.

"Where do you know her from?"

"I know her from a house I had worked on."

"So you get a little side hustle fixing houses and then start cheating? Take me to her! I wanna know who she is!"

I made Sean take me to her house. We walked on her porch and Sean knocked on the door.

"Who is it?" she yelled from inside the house.

"It's Sean!" Then she looked out of the curtains and saw me standing there.

"Oh shit!" she yelled before she opened the door.

When she let us in, my whole world fell apart. I was crying and everything as I looked into the eyes of the woman he was cheating on me with. I really thought everything was okay between me and Sean. We weren't arguing or fighting at that time. We just had a new baby and the Lord had spared my life. I really thought everything was good. But all along, he was cheating on me with this woman.

The woman had to be a size two. She had short, thin, black hair and looked just like a man. A crackhead man. She looked way worse out of her work clothes. And just looking at her, I asked myself, *is Sean gay?* She didn't have nothing on me. I didn't even feel intimidated by her because the beauty just couldn't compare, even though I had low self-esteem. But even with my low self-esteem, I had to ask, *you wanna cheat on me with this? If you want to cheat on me, don't go from something good to worse! Go from something good to better! Don't just go and fuck any damn thing!*

I told Antoinette who I was. She started apologizing and told me she was sorry about everything.

"My problem's not with you. He made a commitment to me, not you. But I just wanted to be aware of you to make sure you're not somebody I'm letting come into my home or be around my kids."

When I asked her how long had they been seeing each other, the two of them were trying to get their dates together. They were looking at each other and trying to give eye signals and little crazy shit. But she was lying and he was still lying. Every time I asked a question, they gave each other eye signals. Then, I just got up and walked out of the door and Sean followed behind me.

I didn't even get back in the car. Instead, I walked down 7 Mile Road as Sean slowly drove alongside me with the kids in the back seat.

"Bianca, get back in the car," he constantly begged.

"No, just go. I'll walk to the house, just go away."

"Baby I'm sorry, Bianca please, I'm sorry!"

"Leave me alone Sean."

I couldn't even call anybody and tell them about the bullshit situation. I eventually went back home feeling like shit. That same night, Sean grabbed me by my ankle and started crying.

"Baby, I'm sorry. I know I fucked up. I fucked it all up! I know it's my fault baby. I'm so sorry. You were doing everything right! Baby it's me!"

I'm just a stupid person with a big heart and I forgive everybody who hurt me. When I was a child, I was taught to hide people, like the man who was molesting me.

"No, it's not all your fault," I told Sean.

"Don't say that. It is my fault! I know you won't ever forgive me either. I'm going to leave right now. I'll go live somewhere else!"

"Sean, you don't have to go. I accept your apology." Sean just looked at me then, bust out crying even harder.

"I know you want it to be over," he cried.

"No, I don't. We got through the other stuff, and can get through this… but you have to help me because I'm hurt right now." We were on the floor in our living room as I explained, "I don't even know what I'm feeling right now. This is all new to me and I have never felt nothing like this. It's a different kind of hurt. It feels totally different from domestic violence and child abuse. Sean, I've been betrayed like a motherfucker by you!"

It was a hurt I thought I would never be able to get over, let alone write about. Even though he wanted to leave, I wouldn't let him. I was still trying to be that wife and the person they taught me to be in church.

"No baby, you don't have to go nowhere. Where are you going to go anyway?"

"I don't know. I don't have nowhere to go."

The next day, I called Bishop Duren. That's how we were raised. Any problems we had, we were to go and talk to the Bishops about it. So, that's what I did.

"Where is he right now?" he asked with authority.

"He's in the house," I answered.

"Where are you?"

"I'm outside."

"Tell him I want to see him."

Sean went and talked to Bishop Duren. Then, we had an appointment for the both of us to go. That's when Bishop Duren told Sean about himself.

"You done really messed up," he told Sean. "Look at her! She doesn't deserve that, and she's still by your side! She loves you! Do you love her?"

"Yes Sir," Sean answered.

"I don't think you do! If you really loved her, why would you keep taking her through this?"

Bishop really let Sean know that he had a good wife who stood by his side. "But you just keep hurting her and she's trying to make it work."

And I really was trying hard, but the reputation I had in the church was, "Bianca is mean, she's so nasty, she's got an attitude and will flip the script on you in a minute." But nobody had any idea of what I was going through in my house. Everybody was looking at Sean like, *oh poor innocent Sean.*

Even though I forgave Sean and told him he didn't have to leave, I still felt so unimportant. The words Elder Cooley told me as a child came back to haunt me. "You will never be good for nothing but laying on your back! You'll be a good housewife." I thought to myself, *damn, I'm not even that. I'm not even a good housewife. I must not even be good for laying on my back. I guess I'm nothing.* The depression just slapped me in my face. I was already feeling insecure as hell because he kept cheating on me. And cheating on me for what? I didn't know.

Even though I wanted to, I just couldn't get over the Antoinette Davenport situation and it completely destroyed our marriage. The situation made us argue more than we ever did. At the time, I was heavily medicated and my health was slowly deteriorating. I started taking more pills, not realizing I was becoming a drug addict. Then after a while, the pills stopped working. That's when Dr. Hamrick told me to start taking two of everything. And if I ran out, come and see him and he would give me more.

Through all of the drama, my breathing and general health was concerning me. And since I was on narcotics, I could only get my prescriptions every thirty days. But I was running out of pills before my thirty days were up. I had a breathing problem, not enough medication to last me, and I also had to take care of my three kids. Sean cheating on me and all the bullshit with the church people was having a mental effect on me as well. Plus, my medications clearly said, "This medication may cause mental confusion, memory loss, sensitivity to sunlight, illusions and delusions. If these symptoms occur, follow up with your doctor."

I was doing what my doctor was telling me to do, as far as taking my medication was concerned. Then at the same time, my marriage had completely fallen apart. I was sleeping in my kid's room, on the couch, and on the floor so I wouldn't sleep next to him. I felt like I was just all fucked up. My marriage was all fucked up, including my head, my mind, my heart, my house, and the church. Therefore, I was just completely fucked up.

One day, I told Bishop Duren I felt like I was never going to be the same again. He agreed that I may not ever be the same again. When he agreed, I just put my head down and started crying.

After that, me and Sean started fighting more than we ever did. I was getting slapped around, choked and pushed. Sean was saying things to hurt me and I was saying things to hurt him right back. One day, we were heading to church and Sean tried to push me out of the car right onto the Davison expressway.

One time we tried to take a vacation from everything and went to the outlet mall. And even that was a disaster. We tried to shop in order to clear our minds. But we only argued the whole time there. On the way home, Sean got fed up. He pulled the car to the shoulder of the freeway, then got out and started walking.

He just left me and our three kids sitting in the car on the shoulder of the freeway. I sat there for a while thinking he was going to come back. But he didn't. I didn't even know my way back home. But after a while, I drove off and tried to find my way back. While driving, I saw Sean walking and pulled up on him. “Are you going to get in the car?” I asked him and luckily, he got in.

It was crazy to me. He was the one doing all of the bullshit and trying to make it seem like I was the one causing all the problems. He’d tell me I was why we couldn’t get any farther because I wouldn’t trust him anymore. And maybe that was the truth because I didn’t believe a damn thing he said to me from that point on. But how could I believe him? That’s when I suggested we get tested for STDs. Because he had pussy cum all over him, it was obvious he was fucking Antoinette without a condom.

Sean went to his doctor first. When he came home with his results, I met him at the front door.

“What did they say,” I asked as he stood there with his papers in his hand. He just leaned against the door and shook his head while tears rolled down his face. “What did they say? What do you have?”

“The doctor said I have chlamydia.”

“What? You have chlamydia again? This don’t make no fucking sense! You mean to tell me you don’t ever wear a condom when you cheat on me?”

The doctor gave Sean a prescription and some health kits. Then I went to Dr. Hamrick to get tested. He prescribed me the same medicine because I had the shit too. One night we laid on the bed and had a serious conversation. And that time, we were being honest.

"Remember after we got married, I asked were you cheating on me?"

"Yeah," he answered.

"Why did you lie to me then? Was it the same girl?"

"No, that time it was a girl name Darleen." I just sat there like *what the fuck?*

"Do you remember me giving you some pills and saying I had strep throat? I just want you to see how I've been protecting you, since you might think I didn't want this marriage. But I've been trying to make this marriage work. Even after you gave me a STD, I still didn't want to argue, fuss or fight. I told you I had strep throat so you could take some medication. But the real reason I had the medication was because you gave me chlamydia."

"Why didn't you tell me you knew?"

"For what, so we can argue and fight?" I was looking him in his face. "Sean, I love you."

The things I did to get love. In marriage, I was the same as I was when I was a teenager. I was looking for love in all the wrong places. I wanted love so bad, but Sean didn't. It was like I became a slave to him because I knew he was doing me wrong, and I didn't care. I just wanted to be wanted, even if that meant I had to act like I didn't know what was going on with my own husband.

But everything I was putting up with reflected right back on my childhood when I was told I was never going to be shit. I'm only going to be good for laying on my back. All I'm ever going to be is a housewife, if that. Ain't no man gonna want me." And I guess that's why I put up with all of this mess. It was because I remembered all of those bad words. "You ain't gonna be nothing but a hoe!"

And there I was, in a marriage trying to prove a point. It was killing me daily because I was so determined to what, make this man love me?

# Chapter 10

# Hooked

Me and Sean struggled a lot and we barely made it in our marriage. We were fighting like cats and dogs every day. The medication had completely taken over me. I wasn't myself anymore and I was popping pills left and right. I was mentally confused, straight up addicted to prescription drugs, and I didn't even know it.

There were more pills prescribed to me other than the ones I already mentioned. I was now taking Ativan, Vicodin and several other pills I couldn't pronounce. The medications were really affecting my mind and my ability to think. I was sleeping way more than I normally did. And I wasn't just dozing off during the day. I was sleeping for two, three and even up to four days at a time. I would go to sleep on a Monday, and wouldn't wake up until Thursday. Then, next time I'd wake up, it would be Tuesday.

I stayed drowsy and started having memory loss. I couldn't remember the last time I had taken my medication and would constantly keep taking it. It got to the point where I was taking 160 pills in one day. It may sound unbelievable, but it was happening. I couldn't remember taking them and I was only focused on, "I know I have to take my medication."

Nobody knew it, but I was straight up a mentally ill patient and needed some help.

In June of that year, my family came to Detroit for the church convention and they stayed at our house. Because I was so sick, my brother Derrick would stay home with me and Faith while everybody else went to church all day and night. Derrick told me when we were home alone, sometimes I would stand up, then fall to the floor because I was too high to walk. I would try to get up and cook, but he'd stop me and do it himself. He told me about a lot of things I did and didn't even remember.

My entire body was bruised up from fighting. While my family was in Detroit, they asked me was Sean giving me the bruises? I told them no. And I don't even know if they believed me. But the truth was, I couldn't even remember where the bruises came from. I was always asleep, so only Sean knew how I got bruised up.

I'd get up at three and four o'clock in the morning and go to 24-hour Walmart. I'd drive myself there and not remember anything because I was so drugged. Then I would wake up a day or so later and thank Sean for going shopping for me. "I didn't go to the store. You don't remember? You went to the store by yourself," he told me.

*Wow*, I thought to myself. I didn't even remember putting the key into the ignition or anything. I was blessed because God was keeping me in unseen danger. I know for a fact God had to be driving the car for me.

After that, Sean started hiding the car keys from me so I wouldn't go anywhere. And I have to say that it seemed to work because I didn't wonder off anymore after that. But then he started hiding my pills. And when he did that, we started fighting a whole lot more.

He was hiding my pills while I was an addict and you can't do that. Whenever he hid my pills, I had a fit. "Where's my medicine? I need my medicine!" My body started having a breakdown and I needed my drugs. I was told by a doctor that my body was having a worse breakdown than someone who was on street drugs.

The controlled substances send a signal to my brain and tells my brain to do whatever the pill was made to do. Just take my sleeping for an example. Even if I had been sleeping for five days straight, if I took another pill, my brain would get the signal and it was over. I would go back to sleep no matter if I was sleepy or not. Then come to find out, I wasn't even sleeping. I was unconscious in a coma. And this was right in the privacy of my own home.

You may wonder, *well where was Sean during all of this? What was he doing? Didn't he know if you were asleep for that long, then you needed some medical attention?* But the truth is, I don't think he was fully aware, just as I wasn't fully aware. Maybe he thought I needed to stay in the house and not try to drive around. Whatever it was, we weren't fully aware of how bad it was. But my babies were aware. They would come into my bedroom and try to care for me when they saw me out of it.

I remember a time when I was in the bed and Tina brought me a glass of foggy water trying to make me drink it. "Mama wake up. You been sleep for a long time. You didn't eat for a long time. You didn't drink your water for a long time." She was trying to pour the water in my mouth while telling me this.

There was a time when Tina and Little Keith came in my room after they had made some toast for me. "Is she dead?" they asked each other. Little Keith was breaking the toast and trying to put it in my mouth so I could eat it. Seeing my kids trying to care for me made me try to get up and get off the drugs.

After the medication wore off and I woke up, Sean was nowhere to be found. Even the kids didn't know where he was at. Little Keith was basically caring for me and my other two kids all by himself.

Then, I took a good long look at my three kids. I was shocked at how much they had changed. The last I could remember, my youngest child Faith, I had to carry her around in my arms. But now, she was walking around and talking to me. I don't have any memories of my little baby. Not even of her taking her first steps or saying mama for the first time. I broke down and started crying when I realized I had been out of it for so long.

I guess Sean thought I was going to stay in that condition forever. When he came home and I explained to him what the medication was doing to me, it was like he didn't even believe me. When we had arguments, he called me a drug addict and a junkie. And that wasn't helping the situation at all. He was still hiding my pills from me, and we were still fighting because of it.

"Is this what you want?" he'd yell at me. "You want this? Is this what's gonna make you calm down?" Then he'd pour all of the pills in his hand, open my mouth and try to shove the pills down my throat. I would try to fight him off of me as he would hold me down and try to pour a glass of water down my throat.

He was supposed to be helping me in my addiction but he wasn't handling the situation right at all. He was only making things worse out of his frustrations about everything. I guess Sean also needed help dealing with me and my pill problem. But he never asked anybody for help or advice. He would simply hide the pills.

When Sean would get rid of my pills, I would go back to Dr. Hamrick and he would gladly give me some new prescriptions. If I couldn't wait until the prescriptions were filled, then he would give me some medication in his office to take with me.

One day I told Dr. Hamrick I wanted to come off the medication. He said okay. Then he prescribed me morphine and Benadryl to help ease me off. And with me trying to come off of the medication, my body started going through a lot of changes.

"Doctor Hamrick, I got the shakes. And I'm cold and breaking into sweats."

"Okay, I'm going to give you this shot to help you feel better," he assured me. "Did you drive yourself?" When I answered yes, he told me, "Well, you're going to have to stay here and sleep it off for a while."

He gave me the shot and it knocked me right out. When I woke up, I was in the examining room all by myself, completely naked.

I was drowsy as hell and couldn't believe I was sitting there naked. I looked around the room for my clothes and saw them on the floor. That's when Dr. Hamrick walked into the room. "Oh, you're waking up," he said. Then he quickly gave me another shot. When I woke up again, I was fully dressed.

I knew I had been raped by my doctor. But I was so strung out on the medication he was giving me, I didn't even care. I went back to Dr. Hamrick every time I needed some more drugs. I couldn't stop seeing him because I was hooked on drugs.

# Chapter 11

## 136

**O**ne day, Sean and I had a bad fight over God knows what. And because I was so high off the medication, I can barely remember what happened on that dreadful day. But Sean wasn't high at all, and he remembers everything.

While we were fighting each other over God knows what, Sean had me pinned to the floor. He was slapping my face back and forth as hard as he could with his right hand. During the fight, I went unconscious. Then when I woke up, the paramedics were standing over me.

"Are you okay?" the paramedics asked me with these strange looks on their faces. "We need to take you to the hospital right now ma'am. So please, if you can walk, please come with us."

"Okay, let me say good bye to my kids first."

"**NOOOOO!**" they shouted as I started to walk to my kids' bedrooms. Then, before I knew it, I blacked out again.

I woke up in Detroit Receiving Hospital's emergency room with my arms and feet tied to the bed. I looked over at my arms, then I started screaming and hollering. Emergency staff was already standing over me when I woke up in shock. They tried to calm me down the best way they could, and that was by giving me some more medication. But the more I looked at my arms, the more I lost it.

"What happened to me? I screamed. And that's when I was told… I cut myself 136 times.

My arms, stomach, neck, legs, my right wrist, and my back were all cut up… And I didn't know how it happened. But I was told I cut myself.

"Bianca, do you know what happened?" they asked.

"**NO!**" I screamed.

"We brought you in here because you cut yourself. Do you know you cut yourself?"

"**NO!**"

When I looked at my arms and saw them all stitched up, the first thing I thought was somebody got me and tried to rape me or something. Or maybe I was in a horrible accident? I didn't know what happened. I still don't know what happened. I can only go by what was said to me.

The police report stated that Sean said we got into a verbal dispute. Then he went outside and sat in the car to cool off. When he came back into the house, I was standing there all cut up. That's what Sean said, but the domestic violence unit disagreed with that.

Here's a reason why they disagreed. When they came to the hospital to see me, a female officer told me to never say I cut myself again.

"Miss Bianca, I want you to stop saying you did this to yourself."

"But they told me I did it to myself," I sobbed.

"Hold up your hand." She threw a bean bag at me and said, "Catch." So, I caught it. "Now look at your wrist. Which wrist is cut?"

"My right wrist," I answered.

"That's right. You are right-handed. If you would've tried to kill yourself, you would have slit your left wrist, not the right one."

There was a brief pause so her point could sink in all the way. Then she said, "I'm going to give you an example of what I think happened. Yes, I do believe you and your husband got into a verbal dispute. And I believe somewhere in the argument he lost it. He knew you were drugged, talking out of your head, and could barely function. Then, something you said made him snap. And I believe he was the one that cut you."

"You believe he did this to me?"

"Yes. And after he cut your back and your throat, he just went crazy and cut the rest of your body. Then, he had to cover it up to make it look like you did this to yourself. So, he slit your wrist."

She went on to tell me Sean slit my wrist after he saw I was passed out and most likely dead. He couldn't get rid of my body, so he had to come up with a quick story about what happened. Therefore, he had to call 911. She said she believed he slit my wrist because he panicked.

"The dumb bastard should've slit the left wrist," she said. "He tried to make it seem like you committed suicide to cover up what he did."

Sean gave the police my eyebrow arching blade and told them that was the weapon I used to cut myself up with.

The hospital staff stitched me up while I was still unconscious. They told me what happened when I woke up. After they let me talk to the police, they sent me up to the mental floor. About two hours passed, then they sent me home… same day in, same day out.

When I got home, the Young People's Meeting was going on at church. Sean told me Bishop Duren wanted me to come see him as soon as I was discharged. So, I went to see him as soon as I got home.

I sat in his office all bandaged up in white bandages. There was blood seeping through some of the bandages and I didn't even care. All Bishop Duren could do was look at me and ask what happened.

"I don't know." I answered him in a low voice with tears pouring down my face. "I don't know what happened."

"What happened?" he asked again.

"I don't know?"

"Who did this to you?"

"Me."

"No, No," he shook his head. "Who did this to you?"

"Me." He asked who did it over and over… and my answer was, "I did it. They said I did it. But I don't know? I was passed out. I was pronounced dead on arrival is what they told me."

And all I really know is what they told me. They said I was taken to the hospital on a "code red" because I had lost so much blood.

Bishop Duren gave me some spiritual advice. He told me don't let the Devil fool me and he and the Lord loved me. He also told me we'll get through this… not I'll get through this, but we'll get through this. Before I walked out of his office, he stood up to hug me. And with my bandaged arms, I hugged him back.

"You know I love you," he told me as we hugged.

"Yes Bishop I know."

"I love you." He leaned in closer to my face. "I love you," he told me with his face close to my face. "I love you," he said over and over again, and then he tried to kiss me on my lips.

I pulled back and tried to push away because I was confused. I really didn't know what he was trying to do. But even as I pulled back, he kept hugging me and moving his face closer to my face. I really started to get nervous because he wouldn't let me go and was forcefully trying to kiss me on my lips.

"I love you," he told me one last time just before he finally let me go.

I was a little uncomfortable with the situation Bishop Duren and I were in because I didn't quite understand it. But Bishop Duren helped me out a whole lot as far as my cuts were concerned. He never turned down any of my phone calls, no matter how late I called him.

"No matter what time of day or night, I'm here for you," he told me. And he was there. I don't think he knows it, but he is the only person at that church who knew what was going on with me.

Even the incident with Elder Cooley touching my breast. Bishop Duren was the only person in Detroit I told it to since it happened. I also told him about Elder Thomas and Vic McKeever molesting me, even though he still allowed them in his church. He told me Elder Thomas had molested me because it happened to him. But even still, Bishop Duren has a special place in my heart because he was always there for me when I needed him.

There were times when I absolutely hated myself for doing some of the things I've done. And there were times when I didn't give a damn about what I did. When I left

Bishop Duren's office, I didn't give a damn and I stayed at the church for the Young People's Meeting.

I walked amongst the people like nothing was wrong with me. I wasn't embarrassed or scared and I didn't care about what anybody had to say or ask me.

My Aunt Roslyn from Ohio was at the meeting and she was walking around the church looking for me. Sean had told her I was in the dressing room. So, she came in to see what happened to me. When I unwrapped the bandages and showed her what happened, her face instantly dropped to the floor. Tears rolled down her face and she turned her head away. "Bianca, I can't even look." But for some strange reason, I didn't care what she or anybody else thought. I still went and sat in the church service.

I handled the situation the best way I could. But Sean couldn't accept it when I told him the medication made me how I was. He really didn't want to believe it. He wanted to believe I just all of a sudden started overdosing on pills and that's what destroyed our already messed up marriage.

As time passed, Sean wanted us to get out more and start going to church picnics. I didn't want to go because I was feeling like so small and so unattractive. All I wanted to do was isolate myself. Then not even 30 days after I was cut up, we had another fight. We fought because I was in a rage and wanted some answers about what happened to me.

"What happened?" I shouted at Sean. He was there with me and he's the only person who knows what really happened. Therefore, I wanted some answers! "If I was the only person around you, and you woke up all cut the fuck up, you're going to want to know what happened!"

"We were arguing," was all he said.

"What do you mean we were arguing? What were we arguing about?"

"You started talking about Antoinette Davenport," he told me.

"We've had arguments about her a million times! It never led to nothing like this! What the fuck do you mean I was talking about her?"

I questioned him over and over, to the point where I got mad as hell and started fighting him. I wouldn't even say I was mad as hell! I'd say I was hell itself! I didn't know if he did this to me or not! I was laying in the bed at night with a man and didn't even know if he tried to kill me! So yes, we fought like hell and he didn't make it any better.

"You're crazy," he told me. "You are insane!"

What he said really hurt me because no matter what nobody said, **I KNEW I WASN'T CRAZY OR INSANE!**

Sometimes I told myself I was over what happened to me. I tried to act like I didn't notice the cuts all over my body. I didn't look at them. I tried to forget all about it because I didn't feel like facing it. The whole situation was a mystery to me and I didn't like talking about it with anybody.

There were other situations I got past, like the child molestation and domestic violence I was raised in. But this one, I'm not over it. I even lie to myself when I say I'm over the molestation. I'm dealing with the cuts, and the biggest issue I face with them is not knowing what happened. I don't have a clue. I'm totally blank. No matter how hard I try to remember back to when it happened, I can only remember what was told to me. So, it's like I have to take everybody else's word because I was drugged.

I got a bad reaction out of people whenever they saw my cuts for the first time. After it happened, I stopped going out of the house. I missed an entire church convention, and that was rare for me. When people did see me, it was in the winter season when I was completely covered up. But when summer came back around, it started to haunt me all over again.

When it first happened, I disappeared and popped even more pills. I didn't want to be awake to face myself. I didn't want to see myself in the mirror. When I took showers and baths, I turned the lights off. When I came out to go shopping, I wore sheer blouses with the sleeves coming all the way down to the middle of my palm. Then, I would wear a big watch so the slit on my wrist wouldn't show.

Sean was ashamed of me. And that's because people would take one look at me and say, "Oh she's crazy. She's mentally insane." After constantly hearing about how crazy I was, I became ashamed of myself too.

After a while, I started seeking help from other doctors. But every doctor I saw told me, "You have to take your medicine. When was the last time you took your medicine?" I was trying to stop taking the medication. And sometimes I would get mad and flush the medication down the toilet. Then, I would find myself back in Dr. Hamrick's office getting some more medication the next day.

When I say help was not available, I really mean it was not available. Especially in my case because people were judging me by my cuts. When I went to see different doctors and psychologists, off the top, they would think I was suicidal. They thought I was crazy and insane.

First of all, I was depressed as hell when I walked in their offices. And I couldn't even say one word without tears rolling down my face. I felt hopeless, but I was still seeking help from anybody I could. And they all asked me the same question.

"When did you last take your medication?"

"I stopped taking the medication."

"No, you can't stop. Did your doctor take you off?"

They were talking to me from a medical school point of view and they weren't really trying to listen to what I had to say. Nobody was listening to me and that was so fucked up because everybody was judging me from my appearance. They were looking at me like I was suicidal and everybody was telling me what I didn't want to hear.

"Take your medication. You shouldn't have stopped taking your medication. You have to wait until your doctor weans you off the medication."

I thought to myself, *they must be crazy if they think I'm going to keep taking something they said made me do this to myself. To cut myself 136 times? Or to even allow somebody else to cut me 136 times? Never feeling it and not even remembering it? Is that crazy or is that crazy? Why would I keep taking that? I would be crazy as hell to keep shoving it down my throat.*

Since every doctor I went to was telling me the same shit, I ended up going back to Dr. Hamrick. He was the only doctor who could stop the compulsive reactions my body was having, like the chills and the shakes. He was the only one who was helping my drug cravings. He helped my aches and pains by prescribing me different medication and giving me the shots in his office. He was the only doctor who had a cure after all my medicine was gone.

At first, I was going through a thirty-day supply of medication in three weeks. Then it went to two weeks. Two weeks turned into one week. Next thing I knew, I was taking 160 pills in one day, again. In one fucking day I was literally taking that many pills. But what was I to do? I went to all of the licensed professionals. I went to Bishop Duren. My husband didn't believe me. People in the church thought I was crazy. My doctor was taking his own medicine. So seriously, what was I to do?

When I was cut up, I couldn't feel anything. That's how medicated and out of it I was. Getting cut had to be painful because the cuts were so deep that right now, they look like keloids all over my body. The cut on my wrist was so deep that I don't have any feeling in it anymore. I was told I cut into the nerve.

The doctors at the hospital told me the amount of medication I had in my body when I got cut up was enough medication to perform a major surgery. I had actually taken that much medication and was walking around arguing and fighting with my husband. I could have been shot with a gun and I would not have felt it.

I have 136 cuts on my body, all over my body. The cut on my legs have healed and vanished. But the rest of my body is scarred for life.

And even to this day, people still ask me, "What happened?" If I go to a hospital right now, they'll ask me, "What happened? Who did this to you?" It's like the big mystery, "Who did this to you?" I don't know who did it.

Even after all of the bullshit Sean put me through, I can't even say, *Sean did it! He did this to me!* I can't say it because I truly don't know if he did it. Therefore, I say I did it. But I don't even know if that's true either. So, what was I to do?

# Chapter 12

# Mentally Insane

Sitting around the house and looking at the cuts on my body was affecting my mental health. Plus, I was trying to stop taking the medication at the same time and all of it was too much for me to handle. I needed help coping with all of this. I was out of my mind and losing it. And it wasn't long before I ended up having a nervous breakdown. So, I went to DMC Sinai Grace Hospital for help.

The hospital thought it would be best if they admitted me into mental health treatment because I was so stressed out and depressed about the cuts. And because I desperately wanted some help, I ended up checking myself into a mental institution. I had to agree to being admitted because I wasn't suicidal. Therefore, I agreed and signed the paperwork that admitted me into Oakwood Heritage mental facility.

At the institution, I was interviewed, examined, then asked, "Honey what's wrong?" They didn't think anything was wrong with me, until they saw my cuts. When they saw the cuts, they were like, "Oh my God!" I was put into a room with about twenty-five people who were really insane. But I was there for being suicidal.

The patients there were really gone and there was no help for their conditions. Most, if not all of them were not snapping back to reality ever again. Because I was the sane patient around a bunch of insane people, everybody thought I worked there. They thought I was a new doctor. The staff walked around and asked, "Who's the new lady?" When they found out I was sane, I was moved with some patients who were more in their right frames of mind.

I had a schizophrenic roommate named Carrie. When I first saw her, she appeared to be normal. I realized she had a problem when she introduced me to her best friend who wasn't there. As I stood looking out of our room window, she came over to me and told me my hair was pretty.

"Your hair is so pretty. It's so long. Is it your real hair? Can I play in your hair?"

"I don't care," I told her as I stared out of the window at the real world.

The windows were made for people like me, who were in the state of mind that I was in. I looked at the thick bulletproof looking glass thinking, *they had to know what was going through people's heads when they put these windows in here. That's because it's going through my head right now. If these were regular windows, I'd run straight through it.* That's how angry I was. I was mad about what happened to me and I felt trapped by it. Every day I was there made me want to give up. That's because every day the facility made me feel like the situation was getting worse. I thought, *oh my God. I can't believe I'm in this situation. I'm in a fucking mental hospital!*

I had ten days to be there and prove to them I was better in order to leave. Or, if the staff felt like I needed to stay, they would take me before a judge in a courtroom that was downstairs. Then, the judge would make the decision. I basically signed over my rights when I signed in. They could've made me an award of the State if they felt like I couldn't go home and function properly.

Sometime later after Carrie had been all in my face trying to be my friend, we had to go to the staff desk for our nightly medication. Carrie didn't realize I was standing right behind her as she talked to the staff about me.

"I don't want to go to bed," Carrie complained to the staff.

"What's wrong Carrie," the staff asked. "Why don't you want to go to bed?"

"Because… well, I want to go to bed, but I want to change my room."

"Why do you want to change your room?"

"Because of my roommate."

"Are you talking about Bianca?" The staff member looked at me like *don't say nothing.*

"I'm scared of my roommate."

"You're scared of Bianca? Bianca is a sweetheart. Why are you scared of her?"

"Come here," Carrie used her finger and whispered. "Because she know too much."

"Because what?" the staff member asked making sure I heard what she said.

"Because she know too much. That girl know more then everybody in here!"

What Carrie said did something to me. The insane people even knew I had no business being in a place like that. She made me want to shake myself off and tell myself, *you don't have to keep telling yourself you are not crazy! Even the crazy people who's been in here for years can see that you are not crazy! They're going up to the staff saying, "Get her out of here! She's not like us! She know too much!"*

My doctor in the institution was a short Chinese man. Every time he spoke to me, he never looked me in my eyes. Then after three days, he popped off and told me I was bipolar.

"I feel that you are bipolar and you should take this medication," he told me without looking at me.

"What's making you feel like that? First of all, you're telling me you *think* I'm bipolar, not that I am bipolar."

"You are showing signs of being bipolar. So, I have proof that you are bipolar." He started writing out all kinds of prescriptions and started telling me he wanted me to take this kind of medication and that kind of medication.

"You want me to believe your feelings and let you shove some pills down my throat?" As he kept writing the prescription, I told him, "No."

"What do you mean no? This is better for your mental health."

"First of all, you've talked to me for three days and you haven't looked me in my face. You don't know if I'm black, white or Chinese. All you know is what you have on a piece of paper. How can you tell me I'm bipolar and you never even took a look at me or examined me? You haven't run any tests on me and you want me to accept what you feel? Because you haven't even looked at me, I personally feel like you are not a professional doctor."

For the first time he looked up at me. I guess he was used to people who couldn't speak up for themselves because they were sick. But that wasn't my case. I wanted someone to help my situation, not to continue to shove pills down my throat.

"I believe this medication will help you," he told me.

"I feel the medication will only make me worse," I told him in response. "The medication is the problem. I have chronic asthma and upper respiratory disease. I have a doctor who put me on all these crazy medications and told me it will help me feel better and relax."

"Well, I think you need it."

"I know I don't need it. I have too much medication in me and I want to come off."

"That can't happen because at this point, you're on too many medications. We can't just take you off like that. You would be sick and mentally confused."

"That's why I'm here. If you look in your book it'll tell you. I stopped taking my medication and I flushed them down the toilet."

"Well, you have to take these five medications."

"No."

"Well take these four."

"No."

"Take these three."

"No."

"What about two."

"No."

"One."

"No. What about none?"

"If you are going to be here, then we have to have you on some kind of medication." That was basically to show that they were trying to make some type of effort to help me. "How about a half of pill?" he asked.

I agreed and he put me on half of a depression pill. I took the half pill because I figured it wouldn't hurt me. And by my tolerance level for medication being so high, the half of a pill did absolutely nothing for me.

By my fourth day in the institution, I was ready to go home. The patients were fighting each other and the facility wasn't being run right. They had a couple of staff members on every floor with twenty patients. The women were on one side of the floor, the men were on the other side, and the staff desk sat in the middle. All of us watched TV and ate our meals in the same room and there were so many crazy things happening at those times.

I ended up speaking with a social worker who was sent by the State to check up on things. She went around the room and asked us to tell her something about the facility. She wanted to know about how we were being treated and how the facility was being run. When it was my turn to talk, I told her about the situation with the Chinese doctor. And as I explained, everybody started to applaud. As everybody was clapping for me, she looked at me and took her glasses off.

"Bianca, I'd like to see you after group." After group she told me, "You stand out from everybody else. If nobody else can see it, I want you to know I see it. God bless you for standing up for yourself."

She read through my files to see what was going on with me. And she believed me as far as what I said about the doctor. She said I was an inspiration for standing up for myself in a mental institution and saying I was improperly medicated.

While living in the facility, whenever somebody saw my cuts they said, "Oh my God! Oh Lord! Who did this to you?" I got so sick of seeing and hearing people's response when they saw me. It was tearing me apart and I was so depressed while I was there.

At the facility I decided I wanted out of my marriage. That was because I had time to sit back and examine my life up until that point. I asked myself, "How did I get here? How in the hell did I get here? Out of all the places in the world, Bianca, you are here! What the hell?"

When I thought about me being there, it all reflected on my husband. When I went to one-on-one counseling, we reflected on my husband.

"I understand what you are trying to do by coming off the medication," the counselor explained to me. "But the first thing you need to do is get rid of the man who is causing you the stress and acute asthma attacks." I found out some of my asthma attacks were actually panic attacks caused by him cheating and fighting me.

I listened to a lot of the advice the counselor gave me. After that, I took some more time to think. Then, I came to the conclusion that I was going to tell Sean I didn't want the marriage anymore. Even Bishop Duren told us to our faces, he didn't believe I cut myself up all by myself. We said I did it, but he said he didn't believe it. And if I did do it, Bishop Duren said Sean drove me to do it. He also said Sean drove me to the medication because of the things he was putting me through.

What Bishop Duren told us replayed through my mind over and over about how "**HE**" was the cause. Even Dr. Hamrick told me he was the cause of my asthma. That's when I went to the phone and called Sean. I told him I wanted him to pack his bags and leave. I didn't care where he went. But when I got home, he couldn't be there. And if he didn't leave, then I was going to leave.

I had enough. At that point, I looked at my body and mental state and realized I was the person who back in high school was so beautiful and could sing in front of hundreds of people. "I'm not supposed to be here!"

"No Bianca, you don't want this," Sean pleaded on the phone. "I'm going to do better. I know it's hard for you. I know it's the medication. I'm sorry Bianca." Then I talked to my kids and found out Sean was cheating on me while I was in the mental hospital.

After ten days I was finally discharged. “We hate to see you go, but we’re happy you’re going home,” the staff said. They had gotten attached to me from the conversations we had. “I have a strong feeling I’m going to see you again,” one woman told me.

While I was there, I told them all about Dr. Hamrick. One of them told me, “I don’t know where I’m going to see you, but I know I’m going to see you again. With all of that will power and determination you have, I might see you on TV telling your story.”

# Chapter 13

## Worst Thing I Ever Did

When I got home, Sean had a bag packed just like I asked. Soon as I walked into the house, the first thing I asked was, "Where's your bag?" He was being extra nice to me to the point where it was obvious he was doing it on purpose. He knew it was about to be over and he didn't want to mess things up even worse.

But I wasn't telling him I wanted a divorce. Instead, I was telling him, "Right now, we need to separate. You need to go your way and I need to go mine. If it's meant for us to be together, then one day the Lord will give us back to each other."

And after everything, he still didn't leave! And by me being so damn nice, loving, forgiving and caring, my dumb stupid ass allowed him to stay. But to make matters worse, I also stayed myself. And I probably stayed because I didn't have anywhere else to go. Where was I going to go with three kids and no income? I was a housewife who seemed to be totally dependent on Sean.

So, we both stayed in the house together. Everything went right back to our normal. Meaning, nothing changed.

All of the arguing and fighting stilled continued. So, that's when I went to a women's shelter.

I went back and forth to the shelter at least four times because I didn't have any family I could go to. I also didn't want to put our business out in the church anymore. And because of that, I didn't have any church people who I could go stay with. I didn't even want Yolanda to know. Therefore, I absolutely didn't have anybody. It was just me and my kids, struggling and trying to fend for our lives.

At that point, life was feeling like somebody was choking me to the point of where I couldn't breathe. And the same person who was choking me, was the same person I kept going back to. I was trying to make the marriage work while knowing deep within myself the marriage was dead. And what's dead needs to be buried.

Around that time, Bishop Duren made Sean a Deacon at the church. Because of it, I thought he should've had some type of control over himself. He was getting up preaching about this and that to the Young Peoples Department at the church, and he couldn't even control his own self. But he wanted to talk to somebody else. I used to sleep on the couch a lot and he'd always come in there with me.

"Bianca, you can get back in the bed. I'm sorry. I was wrong. Just be patient with me because I'm going through a lot right now."

Sean took my kindness for weakness. And the more I forgave him, the worse he treated me. I guess he felt like I needed him. Plus, he even told me with his own mouth.

"You need me because you ain't shit! You ain't never gonna be shit. Ain't that what Elder Cooley told you? He was right! You ain't never gonna be nothing! You're crazy and your childhood got you all fucked up in the head! I'm not the one who molested you! I'm not the one who beat on your mama! I'm not the one who abused you!"

"No, you're not the one," I said. "You're somebody who's worse!"

Right after that, I tried to kill Sean by poisoning his food. I took some green rat poison and put it in his green beans after I had cooked dinner. I took the little peas out of the green beans and pushed the rat poison in with a toothpick so he wouldn't see it.

I was sick and tired and I had a numb feeling all over me when I did it. When he sat down at the dinner table, I sat right in front of him and watched him close his eyes and say his grace.

"How much do you love me?" I asked him.

"I love you, but you be tripping sometimes."

"Oh yeah? You love me? How much do you think I love you?"

"Well… I know a part of you hates me for what I've done but," soon as he said, "But," I cut him off.

"Do you ever fear I might one day pay somebody to have you knocked off?" He was getting ready to put his green beans in his mouth. "Or do you think I might even poison your food?"

"You wouldn't do that."

"I wouldn't? Check your green beans. Cut them open and look." When he cut the green beans open, he saw the rat poison. "You better be careful what you do to me."

Sean got up and pushed his plate to the floor. Later that evening, he changed his attitude.

"You know what, if I was in your shoes, I would've left me a long time ago," he explained. "I do understand why you're mad."

Even though he said he understood, we still got into it the next night. He was mad and getting ready to leave the house when I started yelling at him.

"Go ahead and leave! Go to those hoes! Run to them like you always do! It's fine! But I hope you come back and stay here with these kids because I'm leaving too! I got somebody coming to pick me up!" He was getting ready to walk out the door. Then he stopped and came back.

"Oh, you cheating on me? You cheating on me?"

"Yeah, I'm cheating on you to! How do it feel when the shoe is on the other foot?"

"You cheating on me?" With the palm of his hand, he hit a glass picture frame that was hanging on the wall over my head. "You better fucking answer me!" Then he started banging on the wall.

I grabbed the phone and acted like I was calling somebody. But I called the CVS pharmacy. Sean thought I was calling a man. I was happy he was mad and I wanted him to get a taste of his own medicine.

"Okay, you'll be here in a minute," I faked on the phone. "Well, he's getting ready to walk out the door right now so come and get me."

Sean hit another picture on the wall, and this time his hand was bleeding. He took his bloody hand that still had some glass stuck in it, and he smeared his blood all over my face. Then he walked through the house and broke every piece of glass he saw with his bare hand. He was pissed the fuck off. But I was satisfied and happy because he got a taste of his own medicine.

And I was trying to be strong, but I just couldn't do it for long. Because of all the fighting we were doing, I started drinking a lot. Then I started smoking cigarettes, which was something I had never done. I was all fucked up in the head at that point. When Sean would come in the house, I would leave out the door and walk the streets. I started giving up. Then I did the worst thing I could've ever done. I went back to Dr. Hamrick for some more drugs.

At that point, I was taking my narcotics with straight shots of gin or vodka. I was becoming what they wanted me to become, a fucking junkie! "I'm fucking crazy! If y'all say I'm crazy, then oh well, I'm just crazy!"

I gave in because it was only me against the world. And if you can't beat them, then join them. And that's just what I did. I joined in on everything. If you wanted to fight, then we were about to fight. You want to cheat on me, well I can cheat too. You want to lie to me, then I'm about to start lying too. You want to make me feel like shit, then I'm going to make you feel like shit too!

So now it was about even. That's where I was at with it. I didn't give a fuck about his feelings, so our fights got worse. Sean got him an extra phone so he could talk to some woman he was fooling around with. When I found out he was talking to another woman on the new phone, we got into it. He pushed me against the wall. I threw a box of cereal at him. When the cereal hit him, he grabbed me by the neck and started strangling me. I started punching him. And as we were fighting, Tina started running up the stairs screaming and hollering.

We fought from the kitchen to down the hallway. Our daughter Faith was walking around in the way. He punched me in my face. The punch knocked me from the hallway to the dining room and I landed on top of Faith. Then he got on top of me, grabbed me by the back of my head and started banging my head into the floor.

When Little Keith heard the commotion, he ran down the hallway to see what was going on. I'll never forget being pinned down on the floor getting beat by a man and looking into my son's eyes at the same time. My son had one foot in front of him, and the other foot behind him. He was frozen in that position. His eyes were wide open, not knowing what to do. He didn't know if he should help or not because it was his daddy and he was supposed to respect his daddy. But at the same time, his daddy was on top of his mother hurting her.

Little Keith was trapped in the middle. I could see the war going on in his eyes. The vision of him standing there frozen still breaks my heart to this day. And while I was on the floor, I promised myself I wouldn't let my kids be raised the same way I was.

Sean and I struggled on the floor until I was able to get him off of me. I got up and pushed him into the hallway. Then he slammed me into the wall. After that, he pushed me into Faith's room where he slammed me into her wooden baby crib, shattering it to pieces. Right after that, the fight stopped and I called the police while telling Sean, "This is it! I want you out!"

When the police arrived, Sean was gone like always because he's always guilty.

"When he come back, call us again and we'll come get him," the police told me. They saw the bruises all over me. My head was once again busted open and my lip was bleeding all over the place. I had a boot print in my back that was from three days ago. I drugged myself that day and I didn't remember what was going on. I had to ask my kids about what happened.

"Were your daddy and I fighting?"

"Yes Ma'am," they told me.

"What happened?"

"Daddy kicked you down the stairs."

When Sean finally came home, he hid the phones so I couldn't call the police. When he went to sleep, I took the house and car keys off of his key ring. I knew he wouldn't notice them because he had a ton of keys on the ring. I let him walk out the door that next morning like everything was normal. Plus, for extra assurance, I even kissed him on his cheek like everything was okay.

"See you this evening baby," was what I told him.

"Alright, goodbye baby," he told me back.

When he walked out of the house, I locked the door behind him. A minute later, he was trying to get back in the house by banging on the door.

"Bianca, let me in!"

We lived next door to a pair of senior citizens who were also members of our church. He went to their house and told them what happened. When he came back, I still wouldn't let him in. So he walked away and stayed gone for three hours. Then he came back begging again.

"Bianca would you please open the door? Please let me in!"

"Hell no! Let you in for what?" He walked away and came back later. And that time, I didn't even bother going to the door and responding.

I figured he'd be back later on that night because it was October and he wouldn't be walking around all night in the cold. And when night time came, I heard a loud banging on the front door. The knock was so loud that it scared me and the kids. So, I took them upstairs. And as I walked back down the stairs, the banging started on the back door. I didn't even bother to look out the window, and after a while, the banging stopped.

The next morning, I got up bright and early then went Downtown to get a personal protection order against Sean.

When I made it back home, everything was cool. But when night time came, Sean came back.

He banged on the door, but I didn't answer. After a while he stopped. Ten minutes later, the banging started again. This time it was extremely loud. So, I went to the window. I was going to tell him to stop banging on the door so hard or else I was going to call the police. But when I looked out of the window, the police were already standing there with him.

I opened the door for the officers with my restraining order in my hand. The officers who were standing there with him had seen me on several occasions. These were the same officers who had seen me all cut up. One of them had told me I didn't cut myself and to go get a protection order and have Sean locked up.

"Officers, how are you?" I asked. "If you're going to escort him in, then you have to escort me and my kids out of here!"

"What's the problem?" they asked. I explained how we had a fight and he beat me up in front of my kids. And when I finished, the officer said, "Ma'am, he said you have the keys to his car."

"It's not his car. You can run the plate. "The car is in my name," I explained.

Sean bought the car and gave it to me. But now he was trying to take it back and say it's his.

"Why did you tell us it was your car sir," they asked Sean. "This car is in her name. You lied to us." I had already given the officer the keys to the car like, *go ahead, he can take it and leave. Just don't let him in.* But the officer gave the keys back to me.

"Here are the keys to your car."

"If he's coming in, then I'm leaving out." I held up my protection order like it was a trophy. "If he come in, I have to leave out."

"They can stay," Sean all of a sudden decided. Sean walked away and the kids and I stayed in the house.

After that we were on our own. Nobody saw or heard from us for a long time. I had no idea where Sean was, but he kept calling back-to-back. Maybe he was calling so much because for the first time, he realized I'd had enough.

He was gone for two weeks, and that was the longest we had ever been separated. And maybe that was the reason why he was calling me all day wanting to come back home.

"No Sean, we need to stay separated," I explained to him. "I'm not going to live with you and let my kids see us fighting all the time. There's no way in hell I'm going to keep doing that to my kids."

"It's going to be different this time, I promise."

"You said that last time."

Sean left the house in October. And next thing I knew January had rolled around and I still hadn't seen him. And at that point, I think I was beyond a drug addict. I was running through my thirty-day supply of pills in three to four days. I was always sick and throwing up because I couldn't keep any food on my stomach. I had lost thirty pounds and was looking like a skinny crack-head. There was also a rumor going around the church saying me and another Sister were snorting powder together.

# Chapter 14

# Vengeance Is The Lords

My son had started school at the Pentecostal Church of God Christian Academy. That's when I started going to the school and helping out with the other parents. I tried my best to help out as much as I could. But at the same time, I was still a junkie. A Sister who was my friend noticed how I couldn't stay focused on one thought. She would try to talk with me and get me to open up about my problems. "I know something is wrong with you Bianca. I don't know what it is, but I know something is wrong. So, if you need me, I'm here for you."

One day I opened up and started calling the Sister almost every night while I was fucked up and depressed. Besides Bishop Duren, she was the only person who knew everything. My own mother didn't even know what was going on with me.

"Bianca, you need to tell somebody," the Sister told me. But I really didn't tell anybody. I was trying to handle everything by myself and it overwhelmed me.

Then to make my situation even more fucked up, my son got molested in the bathroom at church one Sunday.

Little Keith told me he had to go to the bathroom during service. He was big enough to go by himself. And I sent him by himself and didn't think anything of it. Next thing I know, I was being asked to go downstairs by the usher. Little Keith was in the basement accompanied by Evangelist Hart.

Keith had ran to Evangelist Hart and told him how some boy in the bathroom had molested him. The boy had supposedly gone back up to the church service. We had Little Keith go and point the boy out. Sure enough, the boy was in the service. When Keith pointed him out from the back of the church, we seen he wasn't another little boy. The boy was nineteen years old. His name is Philip Isiah Gillam (MDOC #811973). He had been a member of the Pentecostal Church of God his whole life.

I was furious and wanted to talk to Bishop Duren right away so he could do something about it. Sean just so happened to be at church that Sunday. I told him about it and together we called Bishop Duren's house and told him we needed to see him. Bishop made us an appointment for the next day. And when the day came, we were there bright and early.

In Bishop Duren's office, I told him everything that happened at church the day before. Then I told him I wanted to call the police on Philip for molesting my son. I also told him about the violent things I wanted to do to Philip.

"No," Bishop Duren said cutting me off. "Vengeance is the Lords. I'll talk to Philip's father and we'll straighten out all of this."

We left out of Bishop Duren's office feeling assured that everything was going to be handled. Sean went his way and I went mine. A few days later, I got an unexpected visit from Evangelist Hart. I guess Bishop Duren had sent him to check on us.

Evangelist Hart came in and had a seat. I sat on my lounge chair. The visit was concerning the kids enrolled at the Pentecostal Church of God Christian Academy. John and I had enrolled Little Keith in that school not too long ago. But the reason for the visit was to inform all of the parents who had children in grade K about a sexual assault that may have happened to a kindergartener.

What he said hit me right in the heart. I was so hurt knowing somebody may have molested my son at his school. Damn… we had just gone through this at church. I had gone through this when I was a child. But Evangelist Hart assured me nothing happened to Little Keith at his school.

He explained how molestation had been happening in our church for a long time. He said God wasn't pleased with it and we needed to reveal any and all child abusers. Also, if somebody had done something to me, then I needed to reveal it as well.

For some strange reason, I didn't reveal anything to Evangelist Hart. Maybe it was because I was assured Bishop Duren was going to make sure justice was served like he said it would be. But as time went on, absolutely nothing was done about it. And as for Evangelist Hart, two weeks after he visited me, he suffered a heart attack and died. Then, the situation was forgotten about, like all of the other child molestations that happened at the Pentecostal Churches of God in Detroit, Florida, and around the country.

And even though nothing was done about it, did I get up and do anything about it myself? No, I didn't. The reason why, I didn't… I don't know? What could I do? This was my church I was dealing with and Bishop Duren told me not to do anything. He told all of us not to do anything; all meaning the molestation victims who told him about what happened to us.

I told my molestation story to a Sister from Indiana. We were in Detroit at a church convention when we talked in the bathroom.

"Bianca, I believe you," she told me in tears. "My daddy did the same thing to me and my sister for as long as I can remember. That's why he don't live with us anymore. Now he lives here in Detroit. Bishop Duren lets him preach in the pulpit, even though I told him what happened. And now he's just had another daughter with a Sister from Detroit and she knows all about this to."

Our lives were being destroyed by that church but we were blinded by our love for that church and couldn't see it. We've been molested in our homes by church members, in the bathrooms of the church by the church members, in the balcony at the Detroit church, and in the church schools. Every one of us who's been molested has had a wild life afterwards. But everybody blames us for the way we grew up. It's not our fault we were molested at church and nobody did anything about it.

♫ ♫ ♫ ♫ ♫

One night I put my kids to bed. Then, around two in the morning Antoinette Davenport pulled into my driveway. Remind you, Sean had been gone since October. I had drove past her street on the way to some doctor appointments and saw his car in her driveway. So, I already knew he was still messing around with her.

She pulled up in my driveway blowing the horn and screaming Sean's name. I had just got off the phone with the Sister from church and was startled by the noise. "What do you want," I opened the door and yelled. "Sean's not here so get the fuck out of my driveway!"

She pulled out and drove to the corner of the street. By that time, I had put on my shoes and coat and made my way out of the door. It was about two inches of fresh snow on the ground. When I made it to the sidewalk, she turned around and sped past me. She hit the brake at the next corner and did a 360 in the middle of the street, then sped off. I went back in the house and called Sean.

"Look, your bitch is coming over here looking for you! This is the type of shit I'm talking about! Me and my kids shouldn't have to go through nothing like this!" From me screaming on the phone, my kids had woken up scared.

"Mama is Daddy out there?" they asked me.

After I told Sean what I had to say, he told me he didn't know what I was talking about, then hung up in my face. So, I sat on the floor with my back against the wall. I was already messed up because I was a junkie. The first thing I did when I was under pressure was run and pop some pills. I took my pills with some gin. And not long after that, I was just as drugged as I was when I didn't remember driving to the store. But I do remember going into my bedroom and going to bed. But when I woke up, I was in jail.

The police told me I drove to Antoinette Davenport's house and bust out her window with a bad. Then I went into her house through the window and stood over her bed crying. Antoinette said I was asking her, "Where's Sean? Where's Sean? I know he's here, where is he?"

I was in the Wayne County Jail for a week. When I came to my senses, I called Bishop Duren so he could come and bond me out. He told me he would, but if he couldn't make it himself, he would send someone to get me.

While I was in jail, they made me take a psychiatric evaluation. This was when I started to remember what was going on with me. I remember the correction officers coming to our unit to do a shake-down and made all of us get naked. We all took our clothes off. I stood in line as ten female officers all said at the same time, "Oh my God! Look at her!" They gathered around me and said, "Baby put your clothes back on. Who did this to you?"

The reason I was there turned into a totally different situation.

"Miss, we want to help you. Who cut you up like that? You don't have to be afraid. Who did this to you?" But I was all fucked up in the head, so I didn't say anything.

Later on, an officer came and told me somebody was there to bond me out.

"Is it a man named Bishop Duren?" I asked

"It's a young man," she answered.

"Ma'am, his name is Sean, that's my husband. I have a restraining order against him and he's not supposed to be near me. Y'all can lock me back up because I'm not going nowhere with him. Put me back in my cell and I'll wait three to six months for my court date before I go back home with him."

That situation reminded me of the same dysfunctional situation that happened when I was a kid. I had the police officers and my mother right there. But the house was so messed up that I chose the back of the police car. "Put me in back of the police car." I was in the same situation, but years later in my own marriage. "Put me back in my cell." I looked back on my childhood and thought, *what the hell? I can't get away from the domestic violence! I can't win for losing!*

They made me change out of my jail clothes then took me to the lobby. That's when I saw Sean and his father standing there.

"Is that him?" the officers asked me.

"Yeah, that's him!" So, they took me back. I changed back into my jail clothes and went back to my cell. I'd rather stay in jail where I knew there was going to be some law and order instead of going with Sean. I didn't have to fight my own battles in jail because there was going to be some order no matter what.

I stayed in jail and Sean sent his father back to get me. His father was one of the same people who seen the cuts on my body and asked,

"Who did this to you? Did my son do this to you? I understand he's my son, but if he did this to you, then you need to let somebody know."

"No, Sean didn't do it… they said I did it." I told him like I told everybody else.

Sean's father bonded me out and took me home. On the way there he told me,

"You know you were wrong for what you did."

"But if it wasn't for your son bringing this woman into our life, this would've never happened."

"Well, you're right," he agreed.

When I made it home Sean had one of his sisters drop the kids off. After that, I was going back and forth to court for the case I caught. The Court had me mentally evaluated. After the evaluation the psychiatrist said, "This woman is most definitely temporarily insane." I was temporarily insane was how they put it. And after months of going to court, the Judge sentenced me to five years of probation and outpatient treatment for my temporary insanity.

Not long after my sentencing, I had to go to the FIA office to take care of some business. Then God forbid, I had to see Antoinette Davenport while I was there.

"This bitch had to be here," I said to myself.

"I ain't no bitch!" she yelled back.

"You is a bitch! And you a motherfucking hoe too! Fuck you! I'll get your supervisor because I wasn't even talking to you!"

I talked to the supervisor and let her know what was going on and then I ended up leaving. Not long after that, the bitch put a restraining order out against me claiming I came up to her job and harassed her. The bitch even had the nerve to get me and my kids Medicaid and EBT benefits cut off. The company came to my house and took my oxygen tank away because it wasn't being paid for. So I went to Bishop Duren about it and told him I wanted to sue the lady.

"No, don't worry about it and let the Lord handle it," he told me. "Vengeance is the Lord's." So, I did what he said while my kids and I were being treated like shit.

Then to make matters worse, Antoinette Davenport claimed my kids were being neglected. She actually sent some social workers to my house to take my kids away from me. When that happened, I panicked and called my mother.

I told my mother to come get my kids because the State was trying to take them away from me. When I called her, it was Tuesday. And by Monday night, she was at my house. She hopped in the car with Elder Cooley and drove all the way to Michigan nonstop because she was crazy about her grandchildren.

But the social worker came before my mother got there. And when she looked around my house, she told me, "We apologize. We see no signs of neglect." Even though I was drugged, I was still taking care of my kids. When my mother got there, the first thing she said was I had lost too much weight. I was skinny as hell because I was a junkie. But she really didn't know about it.

It was a little after 10 p.m. and my mother and Elder Cooley were sitting in the living room. My phone rang and it was the Sister from church who I was cool with.

"Turn on Fox 2 News," she told me. When I tuned in, the Fox 2 Problem Solvers were doing an investigation on Dr. Hamrick.

"Ain't that your doctor?" my mother asked me. Right then, everybody looked at me differently.

"Man Bianca, we didn't know."

This is how I know there is a God. I was telling the other doctors my medicine was making me sick and nobody would believe me. But there was one man who fought back. This man's wife popped up dead and she was a patient of Dr. Hamrick. He went to the Fox 2 News Problem Solvers and said, "Hey wait a minute, this place needs to be checked out! I took my wife to this doctor, and now she's dead!"

And I know exactly why he took her there. He took her there because she was going through what I was going through. More than likely, Dr. Hamrick pumped her with morphine and Demerol, then he probably raped her. The man got his wife home and she collapsed and died on the floor. Cause of death, overdose of morphine.

After that, I started getting all kinds of help from people. The Medicaid company was finally talking to me when just before they wouldn't. I would call companies and had to have long conversations with the employees. I was on the phone with people I didn't even know, telling them about my situation. They would tell me when they read my book they can say "I know that lady! I remember that lady and the state of mind she was in. It was me who told her, don't give up!" Everybody was encouraging me now. And it was all because my doctor was exposed. I felt so good after that.

It's amazing how something has to be exposed on TV or somebody has to die before someone is helped. Because of a lady dying, I got a chance to get my life back because Dr. Hamrick was being exposed. There's a part of me that wishes I knew the man whose wife died. Because of him fighting back, I got my life back.

It was reported that Dr. Hamrick had lost his license in another state for drugging and raping his patients. Later on, he was found guilty of illegal distribution of controlled substances and was sentenced to four years in a federal prison.

I went to church and testified about everything. And when I say everything, I mean I told it all. I told them about how I was getting up in the middle of the night, driving around, and not even remembering it. I felt blessed and I was truly testifying to the glory of God.

"Lord, I thank you because I could have killed somebody," I stood at the front of the church and cried. "I could have gotten killed not knowing I was driving Lord! They told me I cut myself 136 times and was pronounced dead on arrival, I thank you Lord!"

I know some people may say, *how can you say thank you Lord for cutting yourself 136 times?* I can say thank you Lord because if I was that out of it, I could've sliced my face open, "That's why I thank you Lord!" My children were in the house. And if I was that out of it, I could've hurt my children. "That's why I say thank you Lord! It could've been worse!"

People looked at me and saw all of the cuts all over my body, but it could've been worse. Even if Sean did it, he could've did worse damage. He could've totally disfigured my whole face. But all I have now is my face and it could've been worse.

After my testimony, the church people took it and ran with it. They made the situation so much worse. A Sister got up the very next service and testified, "Well I don't have a story like Sister Bianca. You know, how she lost her mind and all." *What do you mean how I lost my mind and all? I didn't lose my mind!* They were running around the church saying, "Bianca is crazy. Bianca is mentally insane. She's a fruit cake."

I already couldn't get any of the help I needed from the licensed professionals. But damn, I couldn't even get any fucking help in the house of the Lord! They made it worse, when all I was trying to say was, "Lord I thank you." All you could do as my brothers and sisters was go behind my back and say, "She's crazy?" You couldn't see the blessing?

When I got home from church, I fell on the floor and cried to my children.

"I should've never gave that testimony. Do you hear how they talking about me?"

"Don't worry about it Mama," they patted and rubbed me on my back.

So, when I say help was not available to me nowhere, I mean help was not available to me no… where. Somehow I had to find help within myself. I had to want it bad enough to come off the drugs. I wanted to raise my kids. They were the ones' who made me want to get clean enough to know what the hell was going on around me. I wanted to live drugfree because I didn't want them to grow up the way I did. I never wanted to see my kids hurt from child molestation! And that's why I sent my kids to Florida right after that. Thirty days later, I left my home and moved back to Florida myself.

# Chapter 15

# God Forbid, Back Home

**I** knew moving back to Florida wasn't going to be easy. Especially since I had to move back in with my mother and Elder Cooley. Right before I had gotten married, he kicked me and the kids out of his house. And now we were living with him again. As bad as being in his house made me feel, I had to take it because I didn't have anywhere else to go. I'm pretty sure Elder Cooley felt the same way. But he didn't say anything about it. Actually, he didn't say too much of anything to me while I was there. And that was just fine with me.

But I did do a lot of talking with my mother while I was living there. I asked her why she let us grow up around so much domestic violence? And she had the nerve to tell me it didn't happen. Like I was crazy and imagining everything. Then I asked did she know about Elder Thomas molesting me as a child? She told me, "No!" Then she acted shocked like she really didn't believe me and that only pissed me off. It was like she just assumed I went around lying about shit like that.

Sometime later, I even revealed it to my Aunt Donna. I was telling her in a way like, *you don't have to believe me!*

*If my own mother doesn't believe me, then why should you?* I was talking that way because my family is really close to Elder Thomas and his family. Then she told me, "Bianca, I believe you because he did it to me when I was a little girl." What kind of shit is that? And he's still doing it right now!

Elder Thomas has a granddaughter who's the same age as I. Growing up, we used to play together. And right now, she's a full-blown stud. She's thugged out, has a bald fade, dress like a dude and everything. I remember her mother *(Elder Thomas' daughter)* used to come to church faithfully. Then all of a sudden, she stopped coming and I never knew why.

When I was a little girl and was still being molested, I went over to her house for dinner after Sunday service. When dinner was over, she took me on her back patio porch.

"Bianca, has Daddy ever touched you?" she asked.

"No Ma'am," I lied to her.

"Are you sure?"

"Yes Ma'am, he never touched me." I was still scared at that time.

"If he does, you make sure you tell me, you hear?" I nodded my head, not knowing he had molested and raped his own daughters.

Come to find out, she left the church after she had revealed her daddy to her mother. She told on him because even as an adult, he still tried to come on to her. And this was his blood daughter. But just recently, she came back to church and attends regularly.

But the man has been raping and molesting his own daughters: raping and molesting his own granddaughters: raping and molesting other kids in the church, boys as well as girls. And the sad thing is, he's still there like he's done nothing.

I used to just sit in church and pray to God, *Lord, this is your house. How do you let people like this exist and continue to scar and wound young people?* It really made me question my faith in God. I thought, *Lord, how could you let this happen? This is your house and a lot of the situations took place right in the bathroom.*

The victims started confiding in each other. The little boys are grown up now. They would say in their testimonies to each other how Elder Thomas took them into the church bathroom and straight up penetrated them. My friend Roy McDougal, he was one of the victims also. Roy and I were really close growing up. One time I was walking to the church kitchen and saw Roy run out of the restroom. His eyes were red and teary. I tried to stop him to ask, "What's wrong," but Elder Thomas was coming out of the door right behind him.

When it came to Roy, we were told his father *(Elder McDougal)* told Roy, "Tell us who did this and I promise I'll kill him!" Then, he flipped the script and said, "I don't even want to know because I know I'll kill him." Out of all of the boys Elder Thomas was molesting, Roy is the only one I know who's trying to stay away from the homosexual spirit. He's married now and everything. But some of the other gay boys in the church still calls Roy and tell him, "You know you want it. You know you don't like fish." Roy tells them, "Stop calling me, I'm not like that no more. You know I don't do that anymore." But that's a strong spirit to try to fight and I feel sorry for Roy.

Some of the openly gay boys married some girls from Detroit. Now one of them is beating the mess out of his wife. In my opinion, that's the only way he can prove his manhood because his manhood was snatched away from him as a little boy. He was done the same way. He was beat on and that's the only way he feels he could be a man. And I think he'll stay that way until somebody sit him down and let him know, 'what was done to you was wrong.'

Elder Thomas has another granddaughter. Her name is Sandy and we know it's happening to her also. She's just so spaced out. When I came back to Florida, we were in the Bishop's Council convention and Sandy was sitting right behind me next to her mother. And her mother isn't far from being spaced out herself. When I saw the facial expressions Sandy was making, I tapped my aunt on her shoulder and said, "Look at this little girl! Don't y'all see something is wrong? Her granddaddy is touching her too! How can y'all sit up in church and not see this?"

Sandy is about twelve years old now. But even when she was younger, she was having little incidents where she was caught messing around with other kids when she would spend the night at their homes. She was doing a lot of things little kids just wouldn't be doing. And the situation is tripped out because I know it's still happening.

Even with all of this going on, I still went to church every time there was service. I was hoping something would change, that my life would change. I was hoping somebody would preach about that child molester and have him locked up. But nothing ever happened and I started to feel more and more like crap.

Just being there made me feel like I couldn't even trust the people in the "house of the Lord." All of the trust I had in people was gone, and still is. I don't trust nobody. No matter how much I tell a person I kind of trust them, I don't. I'm just living right now, and that's it. I don't trust nobody in my house and there's nothing they can do that will surprise me. I look forward to people hurting me and letting me down. I don't even trust my own mother. And as much as I love my kids, I don't trust them either. I look forward to my kids betraying me because I don't trust nobody.

That's why I stayed to myself. But even with who I am, you think people stayed away from me? Hell no! Even when I told them how I felt when I went to church, they still pressured me to go. Everybody I've ever known was, and still is to this day, a member of that church. Therefore, the pressure for me to go to that church was tremendous.

I tried purposely to keep people away from me and it didn't work. I'd be mean to people on purpose and it didn't work. I became a totally different person and I liked who I became. I couldn't even feel. I couldn't have a relationship with a man because there was nothing there for me to give.

I remember when I was at the church convention. It was winter time and I felt safe because I could wear long sleeves. There was a Sister who knew me. She sat on the side of me and asked, "What happened? The top part of your hand is all cut up. You tried to commit suicide or something? Ha, ha, ha!" I just stared at her with an expressionless face and didn't say anything. By the end of the service she said, "You know I was just joking. Were you in a car accident or something?" Still, I gave her the same response.

People are cruel and don't care about you. It was hard for me to live in Detroit and struggled with this by myself. Now I'm back in Florida, and it's even harder. Then, on top of me feeling like people were cruel, I was also feeling bad because I didn't have any money to support my kids with. Or, a home we all could live in. I couldn't even buy them any clothes. Thank God for the Salvation Army because that's where I went to get help with clothes for my kids.

I had been calling Sean and asking him to send some money so I could take care of our kids. He always told me he didn't have anything. Then he brushed me off. One day I was fed up and told Sean I was going to call and tell Bishop Duren on him and see what he had to say about it. Sean all of a sudden changed. "Bishop Duren can't tell me shit!" Sean yelled. "Call Bishop Duren, I don't care what he say!"

Never in Sean's life had he talked that way about Bishop Duren. I couldn't understand why all of a sudden, he felt as if Bishop Duren couldn't tell him shit? He'd been telling Sean what to do his entire life and Sean never talked back or questioned it. But later on, Sean confided in me and told me he found out Bishop Duren was his biological father.

I know Sean had to have been crushed when he found out Bishop Duren was his father because it crushed me. All of his life he thought the man who raised him was his father. Then come to find out, he isn't. That has to be devastating. It tripped me out because now my kids are Bishop Duren's biological grandkids.

But what tripped me out most, was the fact that Sean was cheating on me with Bishop Duren's granddaughter Crystal Duren, who is actually Sean's niece! He cheated on me with his own niece and he didn't even know it. But Bishop Duren knew about this and he didn't tell either one of them. That was really messed up. Sean was basically like, forget me and Bishop Duren, and he continued to avoid helping me financially. So, I had to fend for myself.

I had to hustle, but I didn't have a hustle. I couldn't even find a hustle. There was only so much I could do, and that seemed like nothing. I couldn't even become a stripper because my body was all cut up. I was too scared to stand on the corner or get on the internet and prostitute myself. Plus, I was also ashamed to let a man see my abused body. The only things I knew how to do was sing, play the piano, and pray. I wasn't even mentally stable enough to go and get a decent job. Hell, I don't even think I could get past an interview.

I was trying to get all the government assistance I could possibly get. But at that time, it seemed like the FIA office wasn't helping me enough. They did provide me with some benefits. But I still needed money to rent a home for me and my kids. So, I went back to asking people for help. And most of the people were church people.

I begged everybody I knew. But the people I knew didn't have much. If I could, I would get a few dollars from this person, and a couple dollars from that person. And then I promised to pay them back when I got on my feet. For three weeks I did this, and I owed out $250. And I used that money to care for my kids the best I could.

Begging people for some money made me feel like a worthless piece of shit. And because I was feeling like shit, I believe it had a tremendous effect on my physical health. My health was going down fast. There wasn't one day where my body wasn't weak, or I was wheezing, or depressed and had a migraine headache. I was in and out of the hospital all of the time. And each time in the hospital, I had to get a mental evaluation when they saw the cuts all over my body.

I was sent to a psychiatrist and I had to go three times a week. It was about two weeks after my first visit when I finished telling him every little detail about my life. After I told him about myself, he just sat there and looked at me in amazement. "I've never heard of anything like this before," the psychiatrist told me. "And the most unbelievable part about this is, your whole life has been messed up by a church. The place where you were going to for help, was the place that was killing you! And it was a church! You should never step another foot back in that place again! Then, you should call the police, the Lifetime movie network, or Oprah Winfrey and tell your story!"

The psychiatrist and I became really good friends. He diagnosed me as being disabled so I could receive some benefits. “Bianca, you are most definitely disabled,” he told me. “I think someone needs to care for you for the rest of your life.” After that, I applied for Section 8 low-income housing and was approved. I thought it was a blessing. Now I had a home I could take my kids to.

But despite what my psychiatrist recommended, I kept going to church because I thought things were finally changing. But the more I went to church, the more I saw how things weren’t changing and the more depressed I got. Then, one day at a big church meeting, I saw Elder Thomas from afar.

Therefore, I stopped going to church. And my reason was, “because there are child molesters there.” I even told my kids we were never going back to that church again. Everybody I knew tried to get me to go back. And I told everybody “No” because there were child molesters there. Everybody I sat down and explained this to, were like…

“You mean to tell me the Bishops know about this and Elder Thomas is still there?”

“Yeah, they know! And that molester is still there!”

I stayed away from the church for about a year and tried to deal with my issues the best way I could. Every so often I got depressed when I looked at my body in the mirror and saw all of the scars. And the summer time was the worst time. I wanted to wear the same kinds of clothes all the other women were wearing. But I couldn't show my bare skin in public. I wore pants and long sleeve shirts no matter how hot it was outside. I had just got comfortable with walking around my kids in a short sleeve shirt. But as for going out in public like that, I wasn't ready for it.

A year of trying to stay to myself had its ups and downs. When times were down, I would always call or go see my psychiatrist. He was my biggest crutch at the time. I even took his personal advice and tried to work on my relationship with my mother. She had been trying to reach me and I had been avoiding her. But my psychiatrist didn't know my mother like I know her. And when I finally did talk to her, I wished I would have never did it. When I tried to get some answers out of my mother about my life, she broke down and told me Elder Thomas was my father.

# Chapter 16

# Daddy

**D**o you know how devastating that had to be for me? I'm twenty-seven years old, and had no idea who my real father was. Then after twenty-seven years, she told me some crazy shit like that! I could've killed the both of us!

After I had completely taken in what she told me, I cursed her out, went into a deep depression, and never spoke to her again. With everything I'd been going through since I moved back to Florida, and plus finding out Elder Thomas was my father, I sought refuge in my medications, again. I didn't even care about being a junkie anymore. I popped pills to relieve myself from all the hurt and pain I was suffering from. I locked me and my kids in my own little world, and even shut out my psychiatrist.

About two months had passed. I was feeling really bad about myself and was deeply depressed. I sought out help again. Bishop Ross had just recently died and there was a new head Bishop at the Pentecostal Church of God name Bishop Washington. I called Bishop Washington and told him I needed to talk to him. He gave me an appointment for that Friday afternoon. I really looked forward to seeing him because maybe he could help me out. The molestation that happened to me was really fucking with my head. And that was one of the things I wanted to talk to him about. And not just the molestation, but the fact that the molester was my father. The reality of it all made me want to kill myself. Then on top of that, I had to look in the mirror and see my body. I was just all messed up and needed some kind of help, any kind of help… Lord please, help me.

When Friday came, Bishop Washington acted like he was so happy to see me. He hugged me and asked me why haven't I been coming to church? I told him everything. And the main reason why I wasn't going to church was because Elder Thomas was there. And when I saw him, it brought back memories. When I finished telling Bishop Washington about what happened to me, he just sat there like he couldn't believe what I had just told him.

"Bianca, don't let the devil fool you," he finally spoke to me. "The Lord loves you and I had no idea this had ever went on."

"But Bishop Washington, all of this happened and Elder Thomas is still here."

"If he ever says anything to you out of the way, then you come and tell me."

"Yes Sir."

"The meeting is starting tonight and you need to be here. You were made a Praying Woman in Detroit is that correct?"

"Yes Sir."

"Do you still have your Praying Woman's robe?"

"Yes Sir, I still have it."

"Then go home and put it on. Come back tonight and let the Lord use you."

I went home still depressed but feeling a little better. Bishop Washington somewhat assured me everything was going to be alright and my help was at the church. So, since I desperately needed some help, I was going back to the same church that caused the problems in my life, the Pentecostal Church of God.

That evening I put on my Praying Woman's robe like he told me to do. It was an all-white robe with a matching white hat. I even told my kids to get dressed for church, even after I had been telling them we were never going back there again because there were child molesters there.

Once my robe was on and my kids were dressed, we all caught a ride to church with my mother and Elder Cooley. I didn't even speak to her during the ride. Then as I sat in the service in my white robe, I started having memories as soon as service began. I think the robe and the service combined triggered it… being molested in the church bathroom as a child. I thought about it over and over. And even though I didn't see Elder Thomas that evening, it was as if he was sitting right next to me in his sweaty wife beater T-shirt.

After about forty-five minutes into the service, I couldn't sit there anymore. I walked out and went into the dressing room. Then I took off my robe. I stayed there for about thirty minutes, feeling a little bit relieved because the robe was off. I even tried to go back and sit in the service. But I just ended up leaving right back out and staying outside until the service was over.

When I got home that night, I was really depressed. After my kids went to bed, I ran my bath water. I got in the tub with my eyebrow arching blade in my hand. Then, I cut myself until my water turned red.

I don't know why I did it. Maybe it was because of how depressed I was about my life. But while I sat in the tub, I didn't feel any pain, not even while I was cutting myself. I cut my legs, arms, stomach, chest and my back… then I sat there in a tub full of bloody water. When I got out of the tub, I called my brother Derrick and told him about what I had done. That next morning, he and my mother took me to the hospital to get some help. And I still didn't speak to my mother on the way to the hospital.

The hospital kept me under a suicide watch for three days. They gave me some depression medication, then sent me home. Leaving the hospital, I was depressed as hell and high off the medication. Soon as I got home, I popped some more pills and cut myself again. After I finished cutting myself, I called my friend Roy and told him what I did.

"Why did you do that?" he shouted in horror.

"I don't know?" I cried. "Sometimes I just want to take a razor and slice my face open. It started when I talked to Bishop Washington. He told me to put on my robe and come to church. When I did it, I couldn't stop thinking about Elder Thomas…"

Word got back around to my family that I cut myself again as soon as I got home. So, they sent Derrick over to watch me. He stayed with me all day and night and never left me alone for one moment. When I went to the bathroom, he even stood by the door.

"What are you doing in there?" he yelled. "It doesn't take that long to use the bathroom!"

"I'm just using it. I'll be right out!"

The next day, Derrick went home to get some clean clothes. He was supposed to come right back. But soon as he left my sight and I was alone, I cut myself again…

# Epilogue

**B**ianca never stopped believing in God. Even though the church was the cause of all the trauma in her life, she still went back. And once again, she became an active member of the Pentecostal Church of God. Until one church convention she stood face to face with her father, Elder Thomas. He was walking out of the bathroom while holding his grandson by the hand.

When their eyes met, they both stopped dead in their tracks. He said with a smile on his face, "Hey Bianca, haven't seen you in a long time. You want to come by my house after church? Haven't had a young lady over in years?" Bianca stared at him for a moment. Then she stared at the little boy. She remembered herself coming out of the boy's bathroom over twenty years prior. The little boy had the same look in his eyes that she had as a little girl. Elder Thomas walked away with his grandson.

Later that night, Bianca felt as if she'd had enough. She had a half bottle of medication sitting on the microwave. A bottle of gin sat next to it. She took the medication and washed it down with the gin. Next, she ran some bathwater. With her eyebrow arching blade in hand, she got in the tub. Bianca sat in the tub and thought about the sad life she had lived. Then, with her left hand, she cut her right wrist.

The next morning, Little Keith had just woken up for school by his alarm clock. He walked into the bathroom and found Bianca sunken down in the bloody bath water.

Bianca bled to death in the bathtub…

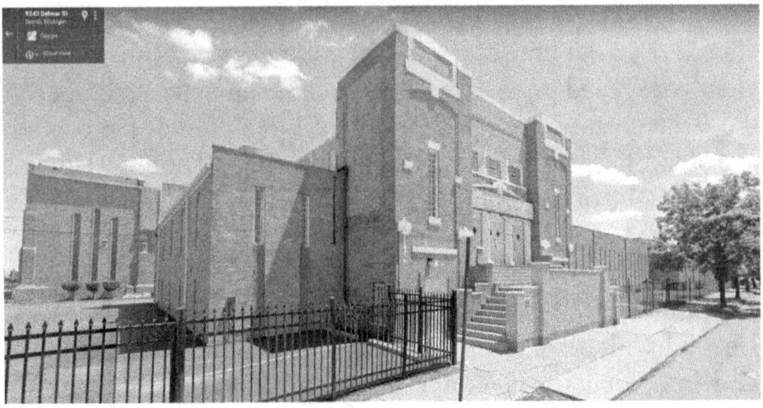

The Pentecostal Church of God (PCG)
9244 Delmar Detroit, Michigan 48211

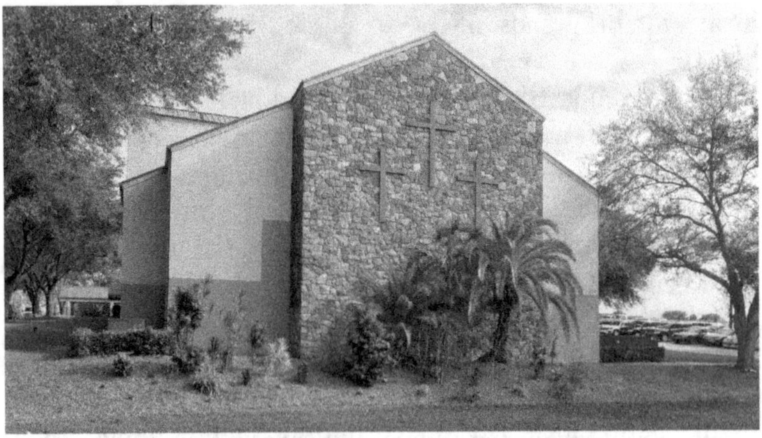

The Pentecostal Church of God (PCG)
2540 Lucerne Park Road Winter Haven, Florida 33881

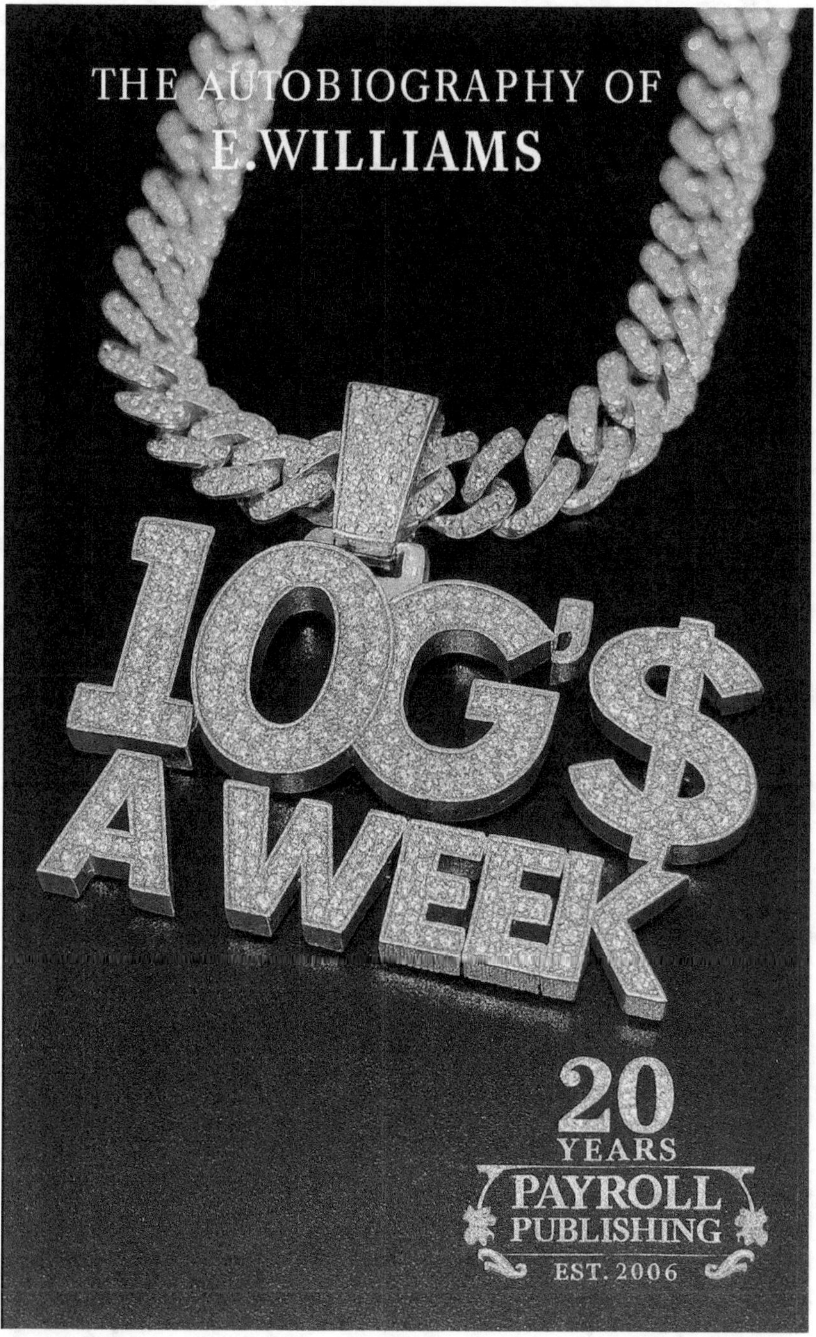
THE AUTOBIOGRAPHY OF
E.WILLIAMS
10G'$
A WEEK
20
YEARS
PAYROLL
PUBLISHING
EST. 2006

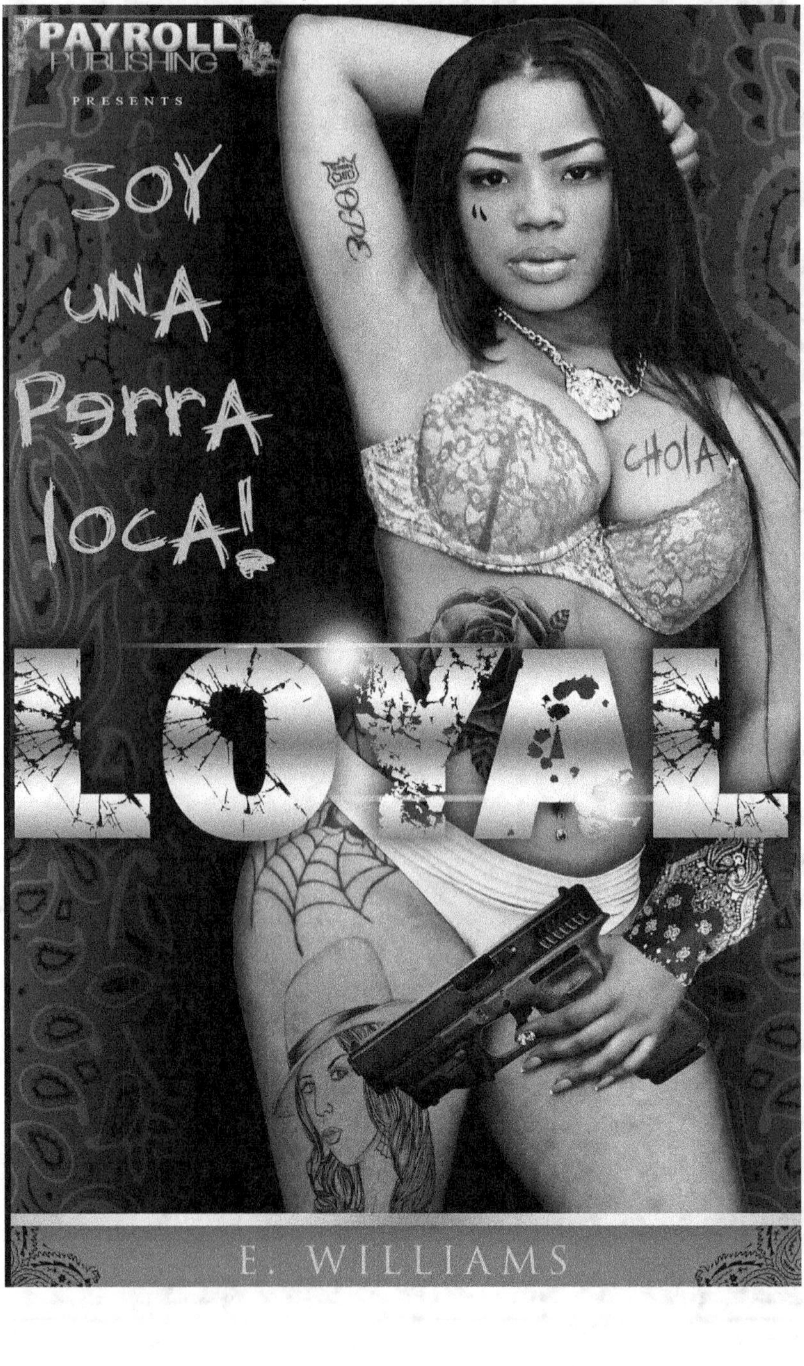
PAYROLL PUBLISHING
PRESENTS
SOY UNA PERRA LOCA!
LOYAL
E. WILLIAMS

www.ingramcontent.com/pod-product-compliance
Lightning Source LLC
LaVergne TN
LVHW052324200926
848481LV00002B/664

* 9 7 9 8 2 3 2 1 8 4 7 3 5 *